PROMOTING *Health* at the COMMUNITY LEVEL

PROMOTING
Health at the
COMMUNITY LEVEL

Editors

DOUGLAS V. EASTERLING
University of North Carolina

KAIA M. GALLAGHER
Center for Research Strategies

DORA G. LODWICK
REFT Institute

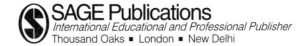
SAGE Publications
International Educational and Professional Publisher
Thousand Oaks ■ London ■ New Delhi

For information:

Sage Publications, Inc.
2455 Teller Road
Thousand Oaks, California 91320
E-mail: order@sagepub.com

Sage Publications Ltd.
6 Bonhill Street
London EC2A 4PU
United Kingdom

Sage Publications India Pvt. Ltd.
B-42, Panchsheel Enclave
Post Box 4109
New Delhi 110 017 India

Printed in the United States of America

Library of Congress Cataloging-in-Publication Data

Promoting health at the community level / edited by Douglas V.
Easterling, Kaia M. Gallagher, Dora G. Lodwick.
    p. cm.
ISBN 0-7619-2262-8 (Cloth)
    1. Health education. 2. Health promotion. 3. Community health services.
I. Easterling, Douglas. II. Gallagher, Kaia. III. Lodwick, Dora G.
RA440.5.P76 2003
613—dc21
2003006025

03 04 05 06 10 9 8 7 6 5 4 3 2 1

Acquisitions Editor:	Al Bruckner
Editorial Assistant:	MaryAnn Vail
Production Editor:	Sanford J. Robinson
Copy Editor:	D. J. Peck
Typesetter:	C&M Digitals (P) Ltd.
Proofreader:	Desiree Dreeuws
Indexer:	Julie Grayson
Cover Designer:	Janet Foulger

Contents

Foreword

Grantmaking foundations in the United States have traditionally played a leadership role in developing and testing innovative ways to improve the human condition. Similarly, since its inception in 1985, The Colorado Trust has employed a variety of grant-making approaches and philosophies designed to advance the health and well-being of the people of Colorado. For example, some Trust initiatives have tested new program models designed to improve health outcomes such as birth weight and child abuse. Other initiatives have supported community-based organizations in designing and implementing programs to address health issues as diverse as suicide, obesity, violence, and the needs of immigrants and refugees in the state. Still others have been directed at improving policy, both within health care organizations and units of government.

To ensure that Trust resources make a real contribution to the health and well-being of Coloradans, we devote considerable time to planning and designing initiatives. This process often requires that we balance competing interests. For example, in selecting topics for Trust initiatives, we strive to incorporate not only objective health assessment data, but also community concerns. Likewise, in making grants to community organizations, we look for health promotion programs that are justified based on research and those that are a good "fit" for each community.

This book describes both the successes and the challenges that arose in implementing seven of The Colorado Trust's community-based health promotion initiatives. These initiatives supported various community groups (e.g., nonprofit organizations, local health departments, school districts, community coalitions) in their efforts to prevent teen pregnancy, improve home visitation programs and school-based health education, address the Healthy People 2000 objectives, maintain seniors in independent-living situations, and promote community health, broadly defined.

Although this book describes initiatives that were designed and funded by The Colorado Trust, it was not written by Trust staff or under the direction of the foundation. Each of the seven case studies was written by a team of independent evaluators. The Colorado Trust highly values evaluation of its initiatives in order to assess the effectiveness of its grant making. We hope that other funders, as well as individuals and organizations operating at the community level, will gain insights that improve their own practice.

In reflecting on our experiences with the community-based approach to health promotion, we believe that there are significant opportunities and critical challenges. On the one hand, we have seen a number of our grantees make significant progress in addressing health issues in their communities. Indeed, many of these organizations and individuals have established themselves as leaders at the local, state, and even national levels. On the other hand, the community-based approach calls for considerable flexibility and patience on the part of a funder, particularly with regard to achieving measurable improvements in health status.

Clearly, supporting communities in their own problem solving has strengths and limitations. We have come to believe that the best approach to promoting health is to combine community-based initiatives with a variety of other strategies that lead to outcomes such as more effective program models, more efficient and equitable systems of health care delivery, more appropriate health policy, and improved living conditions. Only by assembling a diverse portfolio of mutually reinforcing approaches can a funder—and a community— hope to make significant, lasting progress in improving people's health.

Findings from the evaluations of all past Trust initiatives—including the seven profiled in this book—help shape future initiatives of the foundation. We encourage readers of this book to browse through our Web site (www. coloradotrust.org) for a current perspective on The Trust's grantmaking efforts.

—*John R. Moran, Jr.*

Acknowledgments

This book brings together the evaluation findings from seven community-based health promotion initiatives developed and funded by The Colorado Trust in the 1990s. It goes without saying that the evaluators would have had nothing to write about were it not for all the hard work carried out by the organizations and individuals involved in these initiatives.

More than 150 groups throughout Colorado (nonprofit organizations, coalitions, government agencies) received funding from the foundation across the seven initiatives. These grant-funded organizations have included many, many individuals who taught us what community-based health promotion looks like (and should look like) in practice. To each of you, we commend you for the leadership and commitment that you brought to your projects, and we thank you for your openness and candor in sharing your experiences with your individual evaluators. We hope that you will recognize your accomplishments, struggles, and lessons in the chapters that follow.

Supporting the work of the grantees were a variety of managing agencies, including the the Center for Public-Private Sector Cooperation at the University of Colorado at Denver, Colorado Action for Healthy People, the Colorado Rural Health Center, the Kempe Prevention Center for Family and Child Health, the National Civic League, OMNI Institute, and the Rocky Mountain Center for Health Promotion and Education. We would like to acknowledge the staff of these organizations for contributing to the outcomes reported here. In addition, we are grateful for their willingness to enter into the evaluation process as colleagues in discovery.

Obviously, none of these initiatives would have seen the light of day were it not for The Colorado Trust. The foundation invested significant financial resources in the strategy of community-based health promotion, even though this sometimes represented uncharted territory. In addition, the staff and board of the foundation displayed their leadership by setting the vision for these initiatives, encouraging community groups to tap into their underlying potential and persevering with this support as the inevitable real-world complications arose. The following staff members played a distinctive role in the design, management, and evaluation of the seven initiatives included here: John Moran, Jean Merrick, Sally Beatty, Carol Breslau, Nancy Baughman Csuti, Susan Downs-Karkos, Walter LaMendola, Sharon Mentzer, Dana Nickless, and Holly Woods. We would like to express special appreciation to John Moran for his support of the book-writing project (even when it was unclear what the book would say) and to the staff members who provided many useful comments during the review of the manuscript. We are particularly indebted to Jean Merrick for being so conscientious in overseeing this review process.

The folks at Sage have all been amazingly supportive and understanding throughout the entire process of transforming the initial prospectus into a polished book. Marquita Flemming immediately recognized the importance of this topic, affirmed our ideas, and encouraged us through the fits and starts that characterized the early stages. Al Bruckner, who replaced Marquita as senior editor in 2002, provided clear and sound counsel at a critical juncture in the process. MaryAnn Vail, Sanford Robinson, and D. J. Peck each brought a high degree of professionalism, efficiency, and wit to the editing of the manuscript and the production of the book.

As with all research, our work builds on the hard work and creative thinking of those who walked the path ahead of us, or in some cases carved out the path. We are grateful to have had the opportunity to talk with and learn from so many of the people who have developed the theory and practice of community-based health promotion. In addition to the individuals who contributed chapters to the book, our thinking has been informed by conversations with Quinton Baker, Marshall Kreuter, Dorothy Meehan, Steve Fawcett, Bob Goodman, Abe Wandersman, Bill Beery, Kristin Bradley-Bull, Pauline Brooks, Christine Lowery, Joann Tsark, Colin Laird, Nancy Wilson, Michelle Sturm, Sam Burns, Marsha Porter-Norton, Susan Eliot, Alan AtKisson, David Swain, Terri Shelton, and Paul Wellstone.

Finally, we would like to acknowledge the many colleagues, friends, and family members who have encouraged us along the way, particularly our respective spouses, Lucinda Brogden, Paul Nutting, and Weldon Lodwick. It is possible to bring complex projects like this to fruition only because we are connected to a much larger web of supportive people, organizations, and communities.

—*Doug Easterling*

—*Kaia Gallagher*

—*Dora Lodwick*

1

Introduction

Kaia M. Gallagher

Douglas V. Easterling

Dora G. Lodwick

C ommunity-based health promotion is increasingly being recognized as an effective public health paradigm for improving a community's overall health. That local community leaders would have a role in addressing public health concerns is not particularly new. What is novel about community-based health promotion, as a defined health improvement strategy, is that it entails a conscious effort on the part of funding agencies to develop programs that recognize local community concerns and that are designed and implemented with active participation from community representatives.

This book provides seven examples "from the field" of community-based health promotion. The examples are from seven multisite initiatives sponsored by The Colorado Trust, a Denver-based foundation that uses a variety of grant-making strategies to improve the health and well-being of Colorado residents. The initiatives described in this book reflect strategies implemented during the 1990s. At that time, the grant-making goals of the foundation were "accessible and affordable health care programs" and "the strengthening of families."

Although the seven initiatives were developed from a common philosophy, they differ in many important respects: the level and duration of funding, the type of organization eligible for funding, the health issue addressed, the planning process that grantees underwent to develop their strategy or program, the approach to technical assistance, and the nature of the network that grantees formed among themselves. These distinctions in how the initiatives were structured and implemented have resulted in interesting cross-initiative comparisons and have provided insights into the outcomes that result under different funding scenarios within varying community settings.

This book presents the story of these seven initiatives, stories told from the standpoint of external evaluators hired by The Colorado Trust to evaluate the overall effectiveness of the initiatives. These evaluations collected information on the processes through which the initiatives were implemented and also assessed their preliminary results. The chapters that describe these results offer unique lessons for community-based organizations and coalitions that are working to improve the health of local residents as well as for funders who are interested in increasing the effectiveness of their community-based efforts. By compiling these seven stories, the book also offers a prism for viewing the complex concept of "community-based health promotion," which is a multidimensional paradigm for redefining the roles of funders, grantees, participating communities, and the residents who will benefit from these efforts. Finally, the case studies delineate the "real world" complications that naturally arise whenever one attempts to create health promotion interventions that engage the community in novel and challenging ways.

Background on Community-Based Health Promotion

MOVING BEYOND STANDARD APPROACHES TO HEALTH PROMOTION

Allopathic medicine has succeeded in preventing, curing, or at least "treating" many severe diseases and disabling conditions, yet those health conditions that are the most frequent cause of morbidity and mortality (e.g., heart disease, cancer, diabetes, AIDS) continue to challenge modern medicine. Health promotion experts now concur that further improvements in health status indicators are more likely to occur when increased attention is given to health promotion interventions that address the precursors of these chronic conditions, including lifestyles, high-risk behaviors, diet, and the more general community conditions in which people live. It is well recognized that prevention efforts cannot be confined to clinical settings. Although health care providers have an important role in carrying out activities such as screening, patient education, and health counseling, they are only one part of a more comprehensive strategy that needs to be deployed.

To maximize the likelihood that significant population-wide improvements in health will occur, preventive services need to become broader in scope, reaching many more individuals than are currently being educated or counseled in clinical settings. Prevention strategies also need to become more effective and culturally relevant, incorporating behavior change strategies that target risky behaviors while increasing behaviors that improve health and promote lifestyle changes. More generally, the social, environmental, and economic contexts within which people live will also need to be more fully addressed and ameliorated. Responding to this ambitious challenge will require multiple actors in addition to health professionals, an array of intervention settings, and a broad-based intervention focus that considers contextual opportunities for change. The seven case studies in this book offer examples of how this can be done.

DEFINITION

Community-based health promotion, as described in this book, is a prevention strategy that moves beyond the traditional public health model to embrace a broader array of settings, partners, and points of intervention. The defining feature of community-based health promotion lies in the role given to community residents and their representatives in setting priorities for health promotion, in determining how these programs will be established, in monitoring progress, and in evaluating results. Building on the philosophies of community development and community organizing, community-based health promotion mobilizes residents and community-based organizations (CBOs) to improve the community's health with strategies that those residents and CBOs perceive to be relevant and sensible.

WHO IS THE "COMMUNITY" AND
WHAT IS THEIR ROLE IN PROMOTING HEALTH?

One question critical to the development of community-based projects is how the term "community" might be defined. For the purposes of this book, we use this term as a concept that can refer to different types of collective experience. Communities can be circumscribed by means of geography, culture, religion, or other forms of group identity; they can encompass all aspects of life in a particular location or can be narrowly focused on smaller groups such as communities of color and school communities. What differentiates a community from a more individualized perspective is the view toward collective identity. The seven case studies in this book demonstrate the varying ways in which communities can become identified as initiative partners. Whereas several initiatives encompassed entire communities (geographically defined), others entailed more specialized groups such as school districts and service providers offering specialized types of services.

A second dimension relevant to defining community-based health promotion is delimiting the role that the community will play in these projects. Traditionally, the community members engaged in public health programs have been given a very limited set of responsibilities. One frequently used vehicle is the advisory board, which is typically created to enhance the acceptance of a project within a community, to increase the availability of community resources to the project, to maximize the project's credibility vis-à-vis community participants, and to strengthen the opportunities for project sustainability after external sources of support have ended (Kreuter, Lezin, & Young, 2000). When the involvement of the community is structured in this fashion, the ability of community members to advise the project team is often limited. By having others predefine the model to be followed and its expected outcomes, community representatives serve in more of a caretaking capacity and may have few opportunities to adjust or refine the intervention that is under way.

A key distinguishing component of the community's role within community-based health promotion initiatives lies in the range of decision-making authority that is given to community participants. Some initiatives that are merely "located" in the community provide funding to local organizations to implement a health program designed by outside experts (e.g., state or federal health agencies, university researchers). These interventions have typically been found to be effective in controlled research settings and, therefore, are assumed to be effective in other community sites. Community representatives are often considered critical to the program's implementation but play a passive role as a conduit for the interventions that have been imported into the community.

A broader role for the community in health promotion efforts was initially proposed 25 years ago at the 1978 World Health Organization's Alma Alta conference, which espoused "the importance of full and organized community participation and ultimate self-reliance with individuals, families, and communities assuming more responsibility for their own health" (World Health Organization, 1978). Allowing local residents to play a significant role in identifying the issues to be addressed, in choosing the solutions, and in designing the approach to be implemented serves to broaden the important role of the community residents within health promotion interventions.

The accompanying text box provides an example of how community-based health promotion can operate when an intervention is totally defined, developed, and implemented by community members themselves.

During the 1980s, residents of low-income, inner-city neighborhoods of Los Angeles suffered from high rates of infectious diseases transmitted by cockroaches. The public health solution to this problem was to institute an ordinance prohibiting the rental of vermin-infested housing. In other words, local government intended to place pressure on landlords to remedy the underlying conditions that produced the health problem. However, the city ordinance was only selectively enforced, and landlords were rarely prosecuted for violations. Thus, those residents without the financial means to hire pest control services continued to suffer higher levels of illness along with the discomfort associated with living in homes infested with cockroaches.

The "solution" to this problem came not from medical professionals or government agencies but rather from a creative community-organizing effort. Local activists researched the issue of pest control and found a cheap nontoxic alternative to the traditional treatments: boric acid. Working with an entomologist at the University of California, Los Angeles, local residents learned how to administer boric acid to eliminate roaches in a manner that was more effective, longer lasting, and safer than the treatments provided by private pest control companies. Moreover, the boric acid strategy was far cheaper than any other approach on the market, not only because boric acid is a highly abundant, inexpensive material but also because the application was performed by residents themselves with "Getz guns" or fire extinguishers.

The key to the success of this strategy was the intentional diffusion of the technology throughout the neighborhoods. Residents were trained in the use of Getz guns only after they had committed to recruiting and training other residents to adopt the technology. In this way, the Community-Based Cockroach Control program not only addressed the immediate health issue at hand but also set the stage for successfully addressing other health issues facing the neighborhood such as violence—by instilling in residents the expectation that they could have an impact and by strengthening the social connections among residents so that they could become a more potent force in promoting the health of the community.

SOURCE: Goodwin, Zinzun, and Reierson (2001).

RATIONALE

In the following passage, Freudenberg (1998) articulates the fundamental argument in favor of relying on community residents as the primary vehicle for improving local health:

Even the poorest urban neighborhood has a dense and rich configuration of human relationships that can provide support, motivation, and direct assistance to reduce risky health behavior and community problems and to improve health conditions. (p. 18)

Elaborating on this premise, we offer some other more specific justifications for involving community residents in the development and implementation of health promotion interventions:

- Local residents and community-based organizations are in the best position to alter some of the most important environmental and contextual factors that influence morbidity and mortality within the community.
- Because communities vary from one to the other, involving community representatives can help in tailoring interventions to local community needs and circumstances.
- Community members are the ones whose health is at risk when lifestyle changes are not made.
- Community members can serve as guides as to which interventions are likely to "work" within a local community context.
- Involving community members can help to create local buy-in for interventions to be sustained over time.

In addition to these direct benefits of more actively involving the community in the design and implementation of health promotion projects, there are important indirect benefits. In particular, evidence is emerging that a community that is more engaged in solving its own problems is actually "healthier" because higher levels of civic engagement have been found to be correlated with improved health status measures (Putnam, 2000). By working together to address local health issues, communities generate more leaders and residents develop stronger bonds with one another (Minkler, 1997). These forms of social connectedness, also referred to as social capital, have been directly linked to levels of community health. Measuring social capital in terms of indicators of civic engagement, trust, and helpfulness, Kawachi and his colleagues found that states with higher levels of social capital had significantly lower overall mortality rates as well as lower disease-specific mortality rates from heart disease and malignant neoplasms. Moreover, the relationship between social capital and mortality remained significant even when the analysis controlled for poverty and income equality (Kawachi, Kennedy, Lochner, & Prothrow-Stith, 1997).

It is this potential for demonstrably improving community health that makes community-based health promotion such an attractive approach. Underpinning much of the current emphasis on community-based health promotion is the emerging understanding that (a) social isolation has a destructive effect on both individual and community-level health and that, conversely, (b) the strength of a community's collective health or social capital can have a positive protective effect on improving health. The seven case studies in this book offer specific examples of how such promising interventions can be implemented.

THE FUNDER'S ROLE IN
COMMUNITY-BASED HEALTH PROMOTION

Although the defining feature of community-based health promotion lies in the role that community-based organizations and community residents play in planning and carrying out the initiative, funders are also a key part of the equation. Most community-based organizations must rely on outside funding to develop and implement health promotion programs. In providing these funds, government agencies and private foundations have options for defining the target parameters of the efforts and, to varying degrees, for specifying how the projects will be implemented.

In addition to providing dollars, funders can provide other resources that allow communities to achieve more than they could on their own. For example, community-based efforts can be strengthened by funder-supported consultants who provide help in areas such as strategic planning, program development, and evaluation. Networking among community-based grantees can be encouraged. Funders can also assist community-based organizations in identifying empirically tested program models that have the potential to make a real difference on the health issues that the community wants to address.

From a practical standpoint, the critical question with regard to the funder's role in community-based health promotion is the following: How can communities and funders work effectively together so that communities are left in the strongest position to make a difference on the health issues that matter the most to local residents?

The case studies contained in this book illustrate a number of different approaches for strengthening the capacity of community-based organizations and residents to develop and implement health promotion programs. Taken together, the case studies allow us to discover what is required to promote community health while strengthening the community's role in this process. More specifically, the book is designed to answer a number of critical questions regarding the role of the community and the funder in community-based health promotion:

- How can community-based organizations and residents take full advantage of the opportunities offered by outside funders?
- How can funders support decision making on the part of community-based groups and residents while retaining an ability to hold projects accountable?
- How can funders form constructive and authentic partnerships with community-based organizations and residents that bring out the best in both parties?

Background on the Case Studies

THE FUNDING AGENCY:
THE COLORADO TRUST

The seven case studies described here were designed and funded by The Colorado Trust, a private foundation established in 1985 from the sale of Presbyterian/St. Luke's Hospital in Denver. The mission of the foundation has been to "advance the health and well-being of the people of Colorado."

An environmental scanning study carried out in 1991 concluded that The Colorado Trust (1992) could maximize its impact on the health of Colorado's residents by focusing its resources on prevention-oriented interventions and by encouraging more broad-based participation in community decision making. The study report was particularly strong in advocating greater civic participation:

> Many participants in this study report that Coloradans are not participating in decisions that affect and determine their future. They feel out of control. . . . Lack of participation or the perception of exclusion appears to threaten democratic values more than any other dynamic identified in this study. . . . Study members see participation as the single most important remedy to the problems discussed in this report. (p. 13)

At its November 1991 retreat, the board of trustees of The Colorado Trust endorsed the idea of focusing on prevention and civic participation in the first initiative to be created during the 1990s. At the same time, the board decided to change from being a "reactive" grant-making body (i.e., responding to whatever proposals applicants chose to submit) to adopting a "proactive" approach in which the foundation would develop statewide grant-making initiatives. Each initiative would have its own specific set of objectives along with a set of mechanisms (e.g., planning models, technical assistance) for achieving those objectives. In authorizing an initiative, the board would define the level and duration of funding that would be allowed for grantees selected under the initiative.

The first initiative developed under this new grant-making philosophy was the Colorado Healthy Communities Initiative (CHCI), announced in May 1992. As described in Chapter 2, CHCI provided up to 30 communities across Colorado with the resources and expertise to carry out an inclusive, consensus-based approach to health planning and then resources to implement their plans. CHCI was then followed by other initiatives, including the six other community-based initiatives described in subsequent chapters of this book. An underlying premise of the seven community-based initiatives was the concept that local residents and organizations are in the best position to determine what was needed to improve the health of their communities and that the appropriate role for The Colorado Trust was to support and enhance their efforts. This philosophy was codified in one passage of the vision statement that The Colorado Trust adopted in 1994: "The Trust believes in the intrinsic capacity of communities to define and solve their own problems."[1]

OVERVIEW OF INITIATIVES

Table 1.1 provides an overview of the seven initiatives described in this book, differentiating them with regard to the overall objective each initiative seeks to address, the number of grantees funded, the role of various community-level players in carrying out the initiative, the level and form of funding received by each grantee, and the duration of the initiative. This section presents a brief overview of these initiatives and their major accomplishments. These descriptions are presented in the same order as the respective chapters.

The Colorado Healthy Communities Initiative (Chapter 2) provided communities across Colorado with funding and technical assistance to carry out community-wide strategic planning focused broadly on "health" as defined by each participating community. Across the 28 communities that completed the planning process, more than 2,500 citizens participated in at least some part of the approximately 15-month process. As a result of this work, a variety of new initiatives were developed to address issues ranging from diabetes to the pressures of population growth.

In the Community Indicators Project (CIP) (Chapter 3), supplemental funding was provided to 15 of the CHCI communities to develop locally relevant indicators that could be used to track quality of life on a variety of factors determined to be important by the participating communities. These indicators spanned factors such as physical health, environmental quality, economic prosperity, and social connectedness. Indicator reports were published and distributed in 13 of the 15 communities, creating a springboard for community-wide conversations regarding how the local quality of life might be improved.

Through the Teen Pregnancy Prevention 2000 Initiative (TPPI)(Chapter 4), representative stakeholder groups were formed to explore the nature of teen pregnancy within their own community and to adopt locally relevant prevention options. Rather than focusing on sex education or access to contraceptives, this community-based initiative structure led the participating TPPI coalitions to institute broad strategies that addressed the underlying developmental issues facing young people.

The Community Action for Health Promotion Initiative (CAHPI) (Chapter 5) provided funding and technical assistance to allow local health departments and community-based organizations to create and/or expand health promotion programs. Although the initiative specified which health

Table 1.1   Summary of the Community-Based Health Promotion Interventions in This Book

Initiative	Foundation's Objective	Grantees Funded Under Initiative	Key Actors in the Community	Funding/ Community	Duration
Chapter 2: Colorado Healthy Communities Initiative	To enable communities to develop their own definitions of a healthy community and to operationalize this definition through implementation plans	29 communities	Representative groups of community stakeholders	$15,500 for planning phase (15 months) + $100,000 for implementation phase (2–3 years)	1992–1997
Chapter 3: Community Indicators Project	To develop valid and appropriate systems for measuring local health and quality of life	15 communities	Representative groups of community stakeholders	Up to $24,000/year for 2 years	1995–1998
Chapter 4: Teen Pregnancy Prevention Initiative	To develop community-specific strategies to prevent teen pregnancy and to develop community collaboratives	5 communities	Representative groups of community stakeholders	Salaries of four staff members + $50,000/year for 5 years	1993–1998

Initiative	Foundation's Objective	Grantees Funded Under Initiative	Key Actors in the Community	Funding/ Community	Duration
Chapter 5: Community Action for Health Promotion Initiative	To increase community-specific capacity to identify and address local preventable health problems collaboratively	48 community organizations	Community-based organizations Government agencies	Approximately $10,000/year for 1 to 3 years	1995–1999
Chapter 6: Volunteers for Rural Seniors Initiative	To develop volunteer resources to retain rural seniors in their homes	34 community agencies	Community-based organizations Government agencies	Approximately $15,500/year for 1 to 3 years	1995–2000
Chapter 7: Colorado School Health Education Initiative	To implement evidence-based school health curriculum	21 school districts	Health coordinators, teachers, and health advisory committees	Salary of coordinator + $3,000–$12,000/ year for 4 years	1994–1999
Chapter 8: Home Visitation Learning Groups initiative	To promote content learning in self-defined group settings to better serve clients	5 groups of agency representatives	Self-formed groups of individual service providers	$5,000/year for 2 years	1998–2000

issues were eligible for funding (e.g., heart disease, violence, smoking), grantees were free to develop locally tailored strategies to address those issues. Despite the challenges associated with implementing these smaller, more focused programs, project participants reported building personal skills and community support related to health promotion.

In the Volunteers for Rural Seniors Initiative (VRSI) (Chapter 6), local agencies were given funding and technical assistance to initiate or expand programs to meet the needs of seniors, allowing them to remain in their own homes. As a result of this initiative, a large cadre of volunteers were recruited in the 34 participating communities, and they in turn provided a variety of needed services, including meals, home maintenance, transportation, adult day care, and respite care.

In the Colorado School Health Education Initiative (CSHEI) (Chapter 7), school personnel and community residents were convened to form health education advisory committees that in turn were responsible for selecting health education curricula to address the health priorities of local communities and to reflect local values. Health education coordinators facilitated the adoption of these curricula within their respective school districts and became health promotion leaders in their communities.

The Home Visitation Learning Groups initiative (HVLG) (Chapter 8) provided an opportunity for professional development and program improvement for agencies providing home visitation services to pregnant and parenting mothers. An outside facilitator helped each of five groups to design and carry out a learning process that developed skills in areas such as program design, evaluation, and data management. Participants became more aware of the strengths and weaknesses of their programs and then took deliberate steps to improve their program models and the ways in which services were delivered. In many cases, the learning groups set the stage for more intentional evaluation efforts.

VARIATION ACROSS INITIATIVES

The seven case studies demonstrate examples of community-based health promotion in which the participating communities were encouraged to adopt knowledge-based approaches, to nurture and promote local leaders, to develop appropriate stakeholder networks, and to create health promotion programs suited to their unique community contexts. The examples are decidedly varied in terms of the health issues to be addressed, the types of community organizations that carried out the work, and the specific health promotion strategies that were developed and implemented. For example, Chapter 7 (CSHEI) describes the work of local school districts to improve school health education, whereas Chapters 2 and 3 (CHCI and CIP) document the efforts of broadly constituted community coalitions working to enhance overall community health. Other chapters, in comparison, demonstrate how professionally based health and social service agencies collaborated to increase the effectiveness and relevance of the services they provide to their local communities.

The variation across initiatives also serves to demonstrate the different options that funders face when setting up an initiative to improve health promotion at the community level. One issue relates to the question as to who in the community is responsible for directing how, where, and to whom health promotion strategies will be established.

A second decision facing funders is how the strategy will be developed. In some initiatives, community-based grantees were asked to identify their preferred model in their grant proposals and were expected to implement this model once grant funding was received. In other instances, community groups were required to follow a particular planning or learning model while given the discretion to develop prevention interventions suited to local community conditions.

OVERALL PURPOSE OF THE INITIATIVES

Although the seven initiatives differ from one another in obvious and important ways, they share a common underlying purpose, namely, to enhance health promotion at the community level. This enhancement was expected to occur through two complementary pathways: improved health programming and increased community capacity, as delineated in what follows.

1. Communities would adopt programs that would be more relevant, strategic, and/or effective than would have occurred otherwise. This improvement in program design and implementation was expected to derive from the extensive program assistance provided in the areas of strategic planning, "best practices" information, technical assistance during program design and implementation, networking among projects carrying out similar work, and support for program evaluation.

2. Grantees and funded communities would increase their capacity to design and implement effective programming as well as to solve health-related problems more generally.

The first of these objectives focused primarily on the immediate task at hand—the development of new and more effective programming to address whatever health issue served as the focus of the initiative. The second objective reflected a longer range legacy, namely, leaving the grantee or the community as a whole with a greater ability to deal with not only current issues but also whatever subsequent health issues might arise.

In a publication summarizing The Colorado Trust's philosophy about capacity building, Easterling, Gallagher, Drisko, and Johnson (1998) defined *community capacity* as "the set of assets or strengths that residents individually and collectively bring to the cause of improving local quality of life" (p. 7). This publication went on to delineate five distinct aspects of community capacity that the foundation identified as the basis for the funding of these initiatives:

1. Skills and knowledge that allow for more effective actions and programs

2. Leadership that allows a community to draw together and take advantage of the various talents and skills that are present among its residents

3. A sense of efficacy and confidence that encourages residents to step forward and take the sorts of actions that will enhance the community's well-being

4. Trusting relationships among residents that promote collective problem solving and reciprocal caregiving (i.e., "social capital")

5. A culture of learning that allows residents to feel comfortable in exploring new ideas and learning from their experiences

To varying degrees, the chapters in this book document the ways in which capacity was developed at the community, organizational, and individual levels through the seven initiatives.

Organization of the Book

The next seven chapters describe the seven Colorado Trust initiatives that illustrate community-based health promotion. Each chapter has been organized to describe the context of the health promotion issue being addressed, the manner in which the intervention is community based, an overview of the initiative in terms of scope and number of community participants, and a summary of the evaluation outcomes.

The final two chapters synthesize the findings and the lessons learned across the seven case studies. By comparing across the different initiatives, general lessons can be derived regarding the appropriate role of the community in different types of health promotion initiatives and relative to varying definitions of "smart practice."

The first of these two chapters (Chapter 9) explores what the case studies reveal about the concept of community-based health promotion. This chapter begins by addressing the question of whether community-based health promotion is truly a singular construct. By considering different vantage points, it explains why disagreements sometimes arise as to whether or not an initiative is "community based." At the same time, this chapter also shows the value of classifying initiatives in terms of a continuum of *community basedness*. Chapter 9 concludes by considering the implications, in terms of strategic approach and evaluation challenges, as an initiative becomes more community based.

Chapter 10 considers the implications of the case studies with regard to the *practice* of community-based health promotion. This chapter reviews effective ways in which to develop and carry out a community-based health promotion initiative, both from the perspective of a community group interested in addressing a local health issue and from that of a funder interested in supporting such a group.

Our overarching intent with this book is to provide experiences, lessons, recommendations, and conceptual frameworks that advance the concept of a community-based approach to health promotion. Much has been written about the value and the ethics of involving local residents in the design and implementation of health initiatives (e.g., Baker, 1999; Kreuter et al., 2000; Novick, Brownson, & Baker, 1999). However, as the following chapters reveal, much remains to be learned about the practical realities that arise when attempting to balance community involvement against other competing objectives such as program effectiveness, sustainability, and efficiency. Through the lessons provided within this book, we hope to provide a forum through which the opportunities and challenges associated with community-based health promotion can be more thoroughly considered. More broadly, we offer these lessons to inspire others to build on this foundation and further explore the full promise of this innovative approach to health promotion and disease prevention.

Note

1. Although this philosophy undergirds the initiatives described in this book, it should be noted that The Colorado Trust also funded a number of additional initiatives that have been designed to test specific health promotion models in more rigorously defined studies. Examples include Olds's model of nurse home visitation for pregnant and parenting mothers (Korfmacher, O'Brien, Hiatt, & Olds, 1999) and an "interconception" case management program designed to reduce the risk of premature births and low birth weights among women who had previously had adverse birth outcomes (Loomis & Martin, 2000).

References

Baker, Q. E. (1999, Summer). Understanding the community in CBPH. *Voices From the Field*, pp. 1–2. (Durham, NC: Center for the Advancement of Community Based Public Health)

The Colorado Trust. (1992). *Choices for Colorado's future: Executive summary*. Denver: Author.

Easterling, D., Gallagher, K., Drisko, J., & Johnson, T. (1998). *Promoting health by building community capacity: Evidence and implications for grantmakers*. Denver: The Colorado Trust.

Freudenberg, N. (1998). Community-based health education for urban populations: An overview. *Health Education and Behavior, 25,* 11–25.

Goodwin, D. J., Zinzun, M., & Reierson, D. (2001, November). *Presentation of a case study of a successful long-term, community-based, inner-city pest control intervention in Los Angeles County.* Paper presented at annual meeting of the American Public Health Association, Atlanta, GA.

Kawachi, I., Kennedy, B. P., Lochner, K., & Prothrow-Stith, D. (1997). Social capital, income equality, and mortality. *American Journal of Public Health, 87,* 1491–1498.

Korfmacher, J., O'Brien, R., Hiatt, S., & Olds, D. (1999). Differences in program implementation between nurses and paraprofessionals in prenatal and infancy home visitation: A randomized trial. *American Journal of Public Health, 89,* 1847–1851.

Kreuter, M. W., Lezin, N. A., & Young, L. A. (2000). Evaluating community-based collaborative mechanisms: Implications for practitioners. *Health Promotion Practice, 1*(1), 47–61.

Loomis, L. W., & Martin, M. W. (2000). The interconception health promotion initiative: A demonstration project to reduce the incidence of repeat LBW deliveries in an urban safety net hospital. *Family and Community Health, 23*(3), 1–16.

Minkler, M. (Ed.). (1997). *Community organizing and community building for health.* New Brunswick, NJ: Rutgers University Press.

Novick, L. F., Brownson, R. C., & Baker, E. A. (Eds.). (1999). *Community-based prevention: Programs that work.* Gaithersburg, MD: Aspen Publishers.

Putnam, R. (2000). *Bowling alone: The collapse and revival of American community.* New York: Simon & Schuster.

World Health Organization. (1978). *Alma Alta 1978: Primary health care.* Geneva: Author.

2

The Colorado Healthy Communities Initiative

Communities Defining and Addressing Health

Ross F. Conner

Sora Park Tanjasiri

Catherine L. Dempsey

Gabriela Robles

Marc B. Davidson

Douglas V. Easterling

Around the world, cities, towns, and regions are involved in "healthy communities" and "healthy cities" projects. Rather than relying on "expert" assessments of a community's health needs and "expert" models of health care and health promotion, these projects typically involve citizens first defining the important dimensions of health for themselves and then working together with others, including experts, to achieve their visions of a healthy community. These citizen stakeholders are central actors within healthy community projects in establishing goals and objectives and in implementing action projects (World Health Organization, 1995).

Using this model, The Colorado Trust established the Colorado Healthy Communities Initiative (CHCI) to empower citizens to make their communities healthier. Community members, representing all aspects and sectors, defined what a "healthy community" meant for their particular community and then worked together to make their vision a reality. Begun in 1992, CHCI involved 29 different communities in Colorado in a 3- to 5-year process that, within each community, involved strategic planning followed by action project implementation.[1]

The CHCI program was unique in several ways. First, it used a broad, community-based definition of "health." Second, it emphasized participation from and collaboration among many different individuals, sectors, and interests in a community, not only in the definition of health but also in undertaking actions to change community health. Third, it fostered capacity building on both an individual and a group level to facilitate more effective involvement of citizens (Goodman et al., 1998). Fourth, it involved a variety of "communities," ranging from small inner-city neighborhoods to large multicounty areas and from those with homogeneous populations to some that were more ethnically diverse. Fifth, it engaged communities in a community indicator project designed to help them measure and track the health of these communities. Sixth, it included initiative-level, cross-community evaluation planning and implementation from the very outset; evaluation planning began before the program was fully developed, and evaluation implementation started as the initiative began and then continued as each new cycle of the program began with new CHCI communities.

The CHCI processes and impacts are documented in a series of evaluation reports that captured the diverse CHCI experiences in implementing this community-based effort and documented the effects of the projects (Conner, Tanjasiri, Davidson, Dempsey, & Robles, 1998, 1999; Conner, Tanjasiri, Dempsey, & Robles, 1999; Conner, Tanjasiri, & Easterling, 1999). This chapter draws from these reports and ties the information presented there to the larger issues of community-based health promotion and evaluation.

Colorado Healthy Communities Initiative Description

The Colorado Healthy Communities Initiative was based on "healthy city" or "healthy community" programs developed around the world by the World Health Organization and by U.S.-based groups in California, Indiana, and several other locations.[2] These types of programs generally involve a large group of citizens from many community sectors and interests who define health for their community, designate the priorities for action, and then work together to accomplish the results. The Colorado program built on these efforts and extended them in an important way by specifying a set of principles that guided the development, implementation, and evaluation of the CHCI program model.

PROGRAM PRINCIPLES

There are four principles that underlie CHCI: representativeness of participants, consensus decision making, broad definition of health, and capacity building.

1. *Representativeness of Participants.* The healthy communities' approach is anchored in the belief that citizens themselves are the best source of community definition, diagnosis, and action. Because citizens have varying views about their community, it is important to have a broad representation of individuals participate in the process so that the resulting healthy communities processes reflect the views of many people.

Representativeness has two important dimensions. First, communities have different demographic profiles, so representativeness includes individual characteristics such as gender, education, income, and race/ethnic group. Second, communities differ in the sectors or interest groups, such as business, education, environmental groups, and religious groups, that are particularly important to them. These significant sectors, therefore, must also be represented in any effort that truly reflects the community.

2. *Consensus Decision Making.* Participants in the CHCI process (known as "stakeholders") follow a consensus decision-making approach. Everyone's ideas and comments are encouraged during wide-ranging discussions, with the group as a whole reaching consensus. This decision-making approach can be contrasted with majority voting, where a final choice results in winners and losers. In a consensus approach, the decision results from finding common ground among the participants so that the final choice is satisfactory to all members of the group. The understanding among the stakeholder groups is that consensus is a decision that all can agree "to live with," even though not everyone has to agree fully.

3. *Broad Definition of Health.* Another principle underlying CHCI is that participants will adopt a broad definition of health as they decide what a healthy

community means for them. "Health" involves multiple aspects, with a different meaning for each individual and sector in a community. In some cases, the definition of health focuses on disease prevention and treatment such as childhood immunizations and diabetes screening and follow-up. In other instances, the definition more broadly encompasses wellness promotion at the individual or community level such as youth self-esteem building and the development of a sense of community. Some definitions are even broader and embrace a social and political view of a healthy community, including things such as housing, employment, and business development as their targets.

4. *Capacity Building.* As part of its process, CHCI aimed at building both individual and group capacity. At the individual level, participants had opportunities, both direct and indirect, to develop skills in understanding community issues and problems, facilitating meetings, working with diverse groups of individuals, achieving consensus on issues, and exercising leadership in general. At the group level, CHCI project participants developed a group's capacity to work together effectively by defining a common vision, operating rules, and outreach activities that could result in successful processes and products within the group as well as in the larger community.

PROGRAM MODEL

The CHCI model, adapted from the National Civic League's (NCL) model for healthy community work, involved two main phases (Norris, 1993). The first phase, which occurred over 15 to 18 months, involved strategic planning; the second phase was directed toward action-focused implementation activities and ranged from 2 to 3 years in length.

The planning phase had a set of seven well-articulated steps:

1. Provide a catalyst for the project via an initiating committee that then helped to form the stakeholder group.

2. Hold a project kickoff and (re)define "community health."

3. Conduct an environmental scan.

4. Evaluate current realities and trends.

5. Develop a healthy community vision.

6. Select and evaluate key performance areas.

7. Create an action plan.

Outside facilitators, selected by the NCL, assisted each CHCI project as participants worked through the steps of the planning phase. During the implementation phase, communities were generally on their own to implement the action plans they had developed. There was no set of steps to be followed, and the facilitators' involvement was limited.

PROGRAM OPERATION

Small groups of members from interested communities submitted proposals to The Colorado Trust to participate in CHCI. Approval by the foundation provided these "initiating committees" with support to undertake the planning process; on successful completion of the planning phase, the communities were eligible to apply for an implementation grant. During the planning phase, every community received a cash award of $7,500 and facilitation from the NCL (facilitation was funded by the foundation and was valued at approximately $40,000 per community). Each community also had $8,000 available to hire consultants with specific expertise as it developed its action plan (although these funds were rarely used in this manner).[3] During the implementation phase, each community received $100,000 from the foundation along with very limited services from an NCL facilitator.

A total of 29 Colorado communities received planning grants in one of three cycles; of these communities, 13 participated in Cycle 1 (begun in 1993), 8 participated in Cycle 2 (begun in 1994), and 8 participated in Cycle 3 (begun in 1995). Of the 29 communities that started the planning phase, 28 finished it; of these, 27 communities completed the implementation phase. Figure 2.1 displays and lists the 28 CHCI projects that completed the planning phase.

The communities that participated in CHCI were spread across the state of Colorado and ranged in size from large to small, both geographically and demographically. In terms of geography, the smallest community was 2 square miles and the largest was 9,247 square miles. In terms of population, the smallest community had 2,700 residents and the largest had 249,000 residents. Additional descriptive information about the communities and brief community profiles are contained in Conner et al. (1998).

Evaluation Method

The CHCI evaluation had three general goals: to monitor the process of the CHCI program as it was put into operation in individual communities, to identify short-term outcomes for the participants and for the projects, and to investigate longer term outcomes of the projects for the communities.

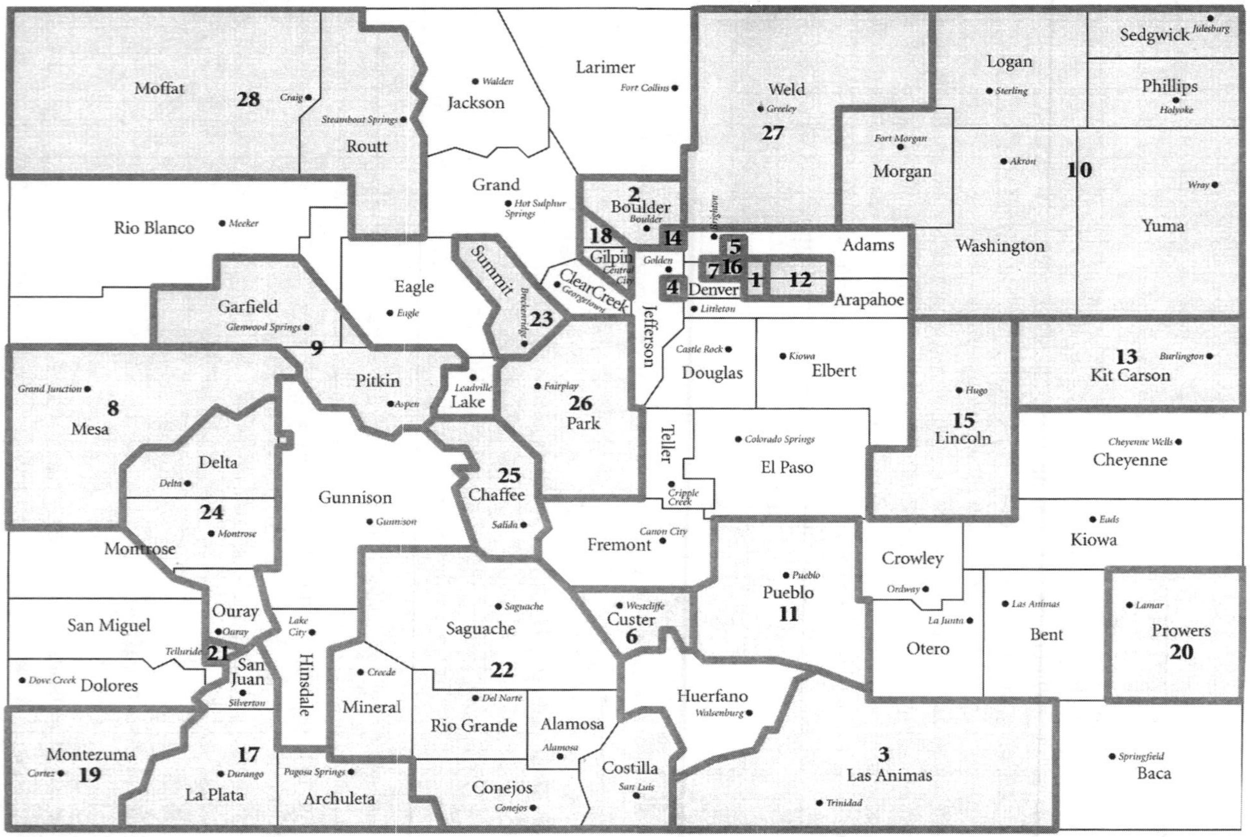

Figure 2.1 Display and Listing of CHCI Projects

Key to the Healthy Communities

1. The Aurora Project (*City of Aurora*)
2. Boulder County Healthy Communities Initiative
3. CHANGE (*Las Animas County*) *now hosted by Fisher's Peak YMCA*
4. Citizens for Lakewood's Future (*City of Lakewood*)
5. Commerce City: Mission Possible!
6. Custer 2020 (*Custer County*)
7. Globeville Community Connection (*North Denver neighborhood*)
8. Healthy Community 2000 (*Mesa County*) *now known as Mesa County Healthy Community Civic Forum*
9. Healthy Mountain Communities (*Garfield, Pitkin and western Eagle counties*)
10. Healthy Plains Initiative (*Logan, Morgan, Phillips, Sedgwick, Washington and Yuma counties*)
11. Healthy Pueblo 2000 (*Pueblo County*) *now known as Healthy Pueblo Communities 2010*
12. High Five Plains Vision for 2015 (*I-70 Corridor—includes the towns of Bennett, Byers, Deer Trail, Strasburg and Watkins*)
13. Kit Carson County Healthy Communities Initiative (*Kit Carson County*) *now hosted by Healthy Living Systems, Inc.*
14. Lafayette Healthy Communities (*City of Lafayette*)
15. Linc-Up (*Lincoln County*)
16. Neighbors Connecting for a Healthy Future (*Northeast Denver—City Park, City Park West, Cole, Five Points, North Capitol Hill and Whittier neighborhoods*) *implementation project is now called Center for Self Help & Development*
17. Operation Healthy Communities (*Archuleta, La Plata and San Juan counties*)
18. Peak to Peak Healthy Communities Project (*Gilpin County and the Nederland mountain area*)
19. The Piñon Project (*Montezuma County, including the Ute Mountain Ute Tribe*)
20. Prowers' Progress to a Healthy Future (*Prowers County*)
21. REACH (*Telluride region*)
22. San Luis Valley Community Connections (*Alamosa, Conejos, Costilla, Mineral, Rio Grande and Saguache counties*)
23. Shaping Our Summit (*Summit County*)
24. Uncompahgre Healthy Communities Project (*Delta, Ouray & eastern Montrose counties and the Somerset area of Gunnison County*)
25. Valley Visions (*Chaffee County*)
26. Vision 2020 (*Park County*)
27. Vision Together (*Weld County*) *now known as Weld Citizen Action Network*
28. Yampa Valley Partners (*Moffat and Routt counties*)

Six evaluation methods were employed to accomplish these goals:

1. *In-depth case studies* were chosen from each cycle to reflect the diversity among the communities.

2. *Stakeholder surveys*, developed with input from stakeholders, were sent to all stakeholders at the end of the planning phase. Nearly 1,100 stakeholders in 28 communities completed the nine-page survey.

3. *Implementation progress reports*, regularly submitted to The Colorado Trust from the communities, were used to assess project activities along the dimensions of participants, actions, and outcomes.

4. *Community leader interviews* were conducted in selected case study communities at the beginning and end of the implementation phase. These interviews were designed to track changes in how the communities made decisions and to gauge the success of action projects.

5. *Comparison case studies* were undertaken in several Colorado communities that were using a different approach to health promotion planning, anchored in a county health department but one that shared the same goal: creating healthier communities.

6. *Community-based indicators* were implemented by a subset of 15 communities for long-term assessment of the impact of CHCI and other activities on communities' health and well-being.

Outcomes From CHCI

An initiative as lengthy, large in scope, and ambitious as CHCI has many outcomes. This section first provides a view of CHCI "on the ground" via a description of the process and outcomes in a hypothetical but representative case, based on the most common experiences in the 28 CHCI communities. The section then describes the major outcomes across all 28 communities in three areas: outcomes from the 15- to 18-month-long strategic planning phase when communities defined health and proposed projects, outcomes from the 2- to 3-year implementation phase when the communities implemented action steps, and two important outcomes that cut across the phases and were unanticipated at the beginning of CHCI.

CHCI IN OPERATION

Every CHCI community was required, as part of the initiative, to follow the general steps in the CHCI model that were described earlier, but each community also was able, with the assistance of its facilitators, to make slight adaptations in the steps to suit the local context. For example, the ordering of some of the steps was changed in a few communities to capitalize on local events or opportunities. These adaptations were not major ones but rather were the types of adjustments that are necessary to adapt a theoretical model, which is intentionally developed for no community in particular, into an operational framework that can guide individual communities. One strength of the healthy communities model is that it recognizes the need for these types of adaptations if the model is to become a living one in the community. Consequently, the model not only permits these modifications but also encourages them.

In the case of the CHCI communities, the modifications in the general model were different in each community. Explaining how CHCI operated on the ground, therefore, would require 28 different stories, and this is not possible within the space limitations of this chapter. Consequently, the description that follows is a hypothetical one of the imaginary community of Mountain View. Although Mountain View does not exist, the description of its CHCI process is realistic in detail, based on an amalgam of the most representative experiences among the actual CHCI communities.

The Application Process

Several Mountain View community leaders first learned about the new program through an announcement distributed by The Colorado Trust. The announcement was not a long one and asked that a group of community members send a brief explanation as to why their community was ready for and in need of a healthy communities process. A group of about eight Mountain View community leaders from various sectors (e.g., education, social services, local hospital, chamber of commerce) sent in an application.

The Mountain View community, through an initiating committee, was asked to submit a full application. (The Colorado Trust directed a few CHCI applicants to take additional action before submitting a full proposal. These applicants either were asked to combine their efforts with those of other applicants from the same community or were encouraged to hold broader discussions with other stakeholders in the community and consider applying for a future cycle of the program.) The full application was focused on who would be brought together to reflect the sectors and interests of Mountain View, what the strengths and challenges were for the community, and what opportunities existed in the community for a process that was aimed at conducting community business differently.

The Preparatory Period

Mountain View received the good news that it was selected to be part of the initiative and that, very soon, a representative from the NCL would be contacting the initiating committee to explain the process in more detail and to assist committee members in taking their first actions. Like all CHCI communities, Mountain View was assigned two experienced and Colorado-knowledgeable facilitators from the Denver-based NCL to work with the community throughout the planning phase of the project. Over the next month, the lead facilitator, Sam, made several visits to Mountain View to learn more about the realities of the community and to explain the steps in the planning and implementation process. He met with the initiating committee, the group that had applied for the program, and focused its efforts on establishing the logistic arrangements for the upcoming planning meetings and on developing the stakeholder group that would be the moving force for the planning effort.

The creation of the stakeholder group was the initiating committee's main task. To do this, Sam and the assistant facilitator, Mary Anne, shared a listing of various sectors/interests and personal demographic characteristics that were typically part of communities or descriptors of community members. This listing included sectors/interests such as business, education, criminal justice, and health and personal demographic characteristics (e.g., gender, age, race/ethnic group, income level). After selecting all of the sectors/interests and demographic characteristics that were relevant for Mountain View, the initiating committee developed a large matrix, with sectors/interests/demographic characteristics across the top and names of community members—about 150 of them—down the left side. This allowed the group to see which individuals could represent which sectors and demographic characteristics. The group then developed a listing of the best set of individuals to reflect the many facets of the community and to compose a group of individuals who would work to accomplish the healthy community goals. The group then set about inviting community members to join the Mountain View stakeholder group, substituting prospective nominees from the master matrix as necessary to assemble a more representative group. Mountain View recruited a group of about 75 potential stakeholders who said they would participate, with a few gaps still to be filled.

The Planning Phase

Mountain View held a well-publicized kickoff for the inauguration of its healthy communities effort. The community had nearly 90 people present, including most of the 75 invitees reflecting many of the sectors and individual characteristics that comprised the people of Mountain View. In addition, there were members of the initiating committee, others from the community who had heard about the event, and members of the local media. The event received good coverage in the local newspaper.

The Mountain View stakeholder group held its first meeting, with the NCL facilitators conducting the meeting, assisted by several members of the initiating committee. The first meeting focused on introducing the stakeholders to the goals and activities for the planning phase specifically and for the entire project generally. The group planned regular meetings, scheduled every 3 weeks from 5:00 P.M. to 8:00 P.M. and usually including a buffet dinner. At the first three meetings, the group began an exploration and discussion of the current situation in the community and the opportunities for change. As with all of the other planning meetings, the group used structured exercises suggested by the NCL facilitators. These exercises included an environmental scan, during which group members surveyed, in an unofficial way, the context within and outside their community; in this scan, they considered social, environmental, economic, political, and other factors relevant to Mountain View. The group also undertook a SWOT (strengths, weaknesses, opportunities, and threats) analysis of the community and held a discussion of the "civic health" of the community, following each stakeholder's completion of the NCL's Civic Index (Norris, 1993). Between these meetings, a subcommittee of the group was assembling a "community profile," using archival data that were readily available to create a picture of the current state of the community. For the Mountain View profile, the subcommittee collected information from the local health department on illness, morbidity, and mortality statistics; from city hall on the demographic composition of the community; from the chamber of commerce on the business and economic situation; and from the police department on several measures of crime. Although the subcommittee's profile was incomplete and selective, it was useful to the stakeholders to develop a better idea about the current realities and to identify areas of community health that might be in need of attention.

Throughout this series of meetings, the group also focused on its composition and structure. The group gave itself a name: Healthy Mountain View. It elected co-chairs and a steering committee to guide the effort and work closely with the facilitators. The group also continued to focus on its composition and to address perceived gaps in the representativeness of the group. In particular, the group believed that it needed representatives from the youth of the community, the poorer segments of the community, and the Hispanic members of the community. The group designated certain people to make contact with other community members who were in these sectors or closely associated with them; the goal was to invite new stakeholders to join the group. After several meetings and only mixed success in adding new stakeholders from these sectors, the group paid less and less attention to this issue, finally deciding to move forward with those who were "at the table"—a total of 49 people.

The group's next meetings focused on the development of a shared vision of what Mountain View would be in 20 years if it had become the healthy community toward which the group was working. Led by the facilitators through a series of exercises, the stakeholders first created a picture of what Mountain

View would be and then prepared a vision statement that incorporated the main aspects of the group's vision. There were five main aspects called key performance areas (KPAs): youth, economic development, education, illness/wellness, and citizenship (in terms of a better-informed and more-involved citizenry). The creation of this vision moved the group to a new psychological level because it was the first concrete product that the stakeholders had produced together and it also established a multidimensional, positive goal for their efforts, albeit one that was in the distant future.

At this point in the process, the Thanksgiving and Christmas holidays intervened and inadvertently caused the Mountain View group to take a short break in its planning because stakeholders were preoccupied with other obligations. Although unplanned, the break served to refresh and reinvigorate the group when it reconvened to continue the next steps in the strategic planning process.

After the start of the new year, the group divided into five subgroups to learn more about each of the five KPAs. These subgroups, each consisting of about 10 stakeholders, worked for the next 4 months to develop statements about the current situation in the area, the opportunities for change, and ideas about possible projects. The larger stakeholder meetings during this time provided opportunities for a review of the subcommittees' work. Several subcommittees worked well together, moving forward with fairly easy agreement among the members. Other committees found planning to be more difficult, with disagreements among members about what the best approaches and projects should be. In one case, several members of one subcommittee who held minority opinions began to disengage from the group, missing more and more meetings and eventually ceasing their participation.

At a major meeting of the full group, the subcommittees presented their plans to the others in the group. The larger stakeholder group wanted more information from three of the subcommittees and asked the steering committee to work with the other two subcommittees to address some overlap in their work plans. After several more weeks, the stakeholder group met again to consider the subcommittees' work and suggestions. One subcommittee (economic development) had not been able to develop its plan fully; in fact, the subcommittee had met infrequently and produced only sketchy ideas. Because of this, the group decided to focus on the other four KPAs.

At this point, a new subcommittee of five stakeholders was formed to prepare the implementation proposal that would be submitted to The Colorado Trust for funding of the implementation phase. It took several meetings for the proposal to be crafted and revised by this subcommittee. With time running out before the due date of the proposal, two members of the subcommittee took over the task of finishing it. After 16 months of planning, the stakeholder group adopted the proposed directions for the action projects and held a celebration to recognize the long hard work by the group.

The Action Phase

Fairly quickly, the Healthy Mountain View group received word that it had been funded for the action phase, with a $100,000 grant for 2 years of work in the four action areas of youth, education, illness/wellness, and citizenship. The steering committee and co-chairs met with the facilitators to lay out the details for the implementation. One co-chair decided to step down, and several members of the steering committee also stopped their involvement. In their places, a former stakeholder and a new community member were added to the group, bringing the total to 12 members. These types of adjustments in the governing group continued over the next 3 years (although planned for 2 years, the project extended the work over 3 years). One of the NCL facilitators continued to work with the group, but only on a very limited basis.

The 3 years of implementation were coordinated by a project director and part-time assistant, both of whom were drawn from the community but had been uninvolved in the planning phase. These staff members reported to the leaders of the stakeholder group. Their work was focused on four primary projects:

- The development of a youth council to work with various sectors of the community on projects of mutual interest
- An after-school educational enrichment program focused on middle school students whom the stakeholders believed were particularly at risk in their community
- A citizen leadership academy to train community members to take more active roles in community affairs
- The development of a special primary health clinic to serve poor uninsured members of the community

By the end of 3 years, the Mountain View community had accomplished nearly all of its subgoals for each of these projects. Three of the projects—the after-school program, the citizen leadership academy, and the primary care clinic—continued after the official CHCI funding period ended, with support from the school system, the city government, the local hospital and physicians group, and a new grant from a local foundation. The youth council was not sustained after the end of the funding.

Although Mountain View was successful in implementing and sustaining most of its projects, it was less successful in maintaining and sustaining the stakeholder group itself. The stakeholder group continued to meet occasionally over the 3-year implementation period, but it did so in reduced numbers. By the official end of the implementation phase, Healthy Mountain View consisted of a core group of 12 citizens, with another 25 involved in secondary ways. The group continued to advocate for its goals in the community, but it did so with reduced visibility.

OUTCOMES ACROSS THE 28 COMMUNITIES

The Mountain View example describes what occurred in one hypothetical but representative CHCI community. In what follows, we describe what occurred across the 28 communities, based on data from the evaluation.[4]

Planning Phase

Large groups of citizens (about 50 on average) came together—and, more important, stayed together—for 15 to 18 months as they worked to define health and plan projects to improve their communities. The majority of stakeholders (55%) reported that they attended all or most of the planning sessions, whereas 21% attended half of the sessions and 24% attended only "a few" sessions. Most stakeholders started their involvement early (71%) and lasted until the final step of the process (74%). Only a small number of stakeholders (13%) dropped out of the process prior to the final steps in the planning process. These data demonstrate the commitment of a number of community members to work together toward community change over a long period of time.

These CHCI planning groups were generally very diverse in terms of community sectors and interests, bringing in those who traditionally had not been involved in health-focused projects such as members of the business and education sectors. The top three sectors represented in planning groups were nonprofits, education, and business, with one third or more of stakeholders representing each of these sectors; parents of school-aged children, government/health services, and environment were not far behind.[5] However, the planning groups were not as diverse in terms of individual demographic characteristics such as age, income, and racial/ethnic background. CHCI stakeholders, based on data from across all 28 communities, tended to be female (60%), middle-aged (71% between the ages of 36 and 59 years), and white (86%); they were from higher income households (46% earned $50,000 or more) and were highly educated (76% were college graduates). The most common underrepresented sectors, based on community stakeholders' assessments, were industry (underrepresented in 19 community planning groups), agriculture (19), legal/criminal justice (17), and health/medical practitioners (15). The most common underrepresented demographic groups were youth under 20 years of age (underrepresented in all 28 communities), Latinos/Hispanics (22), Native Americans (16), and the poorer community members with household incomes of less than $15,000 per year (15).

CHCI community stakeholders defined health in broad terms. All communities easily moved beyond an illness- or wellness-focused view to a perspective that encompassed the underlying factors that determine health, either those focused on community issues (e.g., housing, education, the environment) or those addressing larger structural issues, that is, the way in which the

Table 2.1   Primary Key Performance Areas Across CHCI Communities

Area	Percentage
Issue focused (75%)	
Illness, wellness	13
Education	11
Economy, poverty	9
Environment	9
Families	7
Infrastructure (housing, transportation)	7
Youth	6
Growth management	5
Recreation, culture, arts	4
Safety (crime, violence, abuse)	3
Diversity	1
Structure/Context focused (25%)	
Community (community identity, sense of community)	9
Governance	7
Communication	5
Community leadership	4

NOTE: Total number of areas = 149.

community conducts its community business (e.g., citizen involvement in governance). These latter target areas are particularly noteworthy because they go beyond the types of issues that are the focus of traditional health promotion efforts. In traditional efforts, illness/wellness is usually the central focal activity (e.g., teen smoking cessation); rarely do these efforts include broader issues in the community that might affect illness or wellness (e.g., self-esteem in youth, employment opportunities for youth) or how the community is structured to include or exclude youth in the daily life of the community (e.g., forming a teen advisory council that reports to the city council).

The success of CHCI communities in taking a broad view of health is exemplified in the main components of the communities' visions for their healthy futures. Table 2.1 lists these targets, called key performance areas. Only about 13% of the total set was directed toward illness/wellness; the remainder dealt with topics related either to other community *issues* (62%) or to *structure/context* topics that affect the way in which community work is done (25%). Examples of issue-focused areas would be education, recreation, and transportation; examples of structure/context-focused areas would be citizen governance and intracommunity communication.

In moving from ideas to proposed actions, CHCI groups used consensus decision making. Overall, 81% of the CHCI stakeholders reported that consensus decision making had occurred; in all but one of the communities, the large majority of stakeholders (modal value: 84.6%) agreed that most decisions were by consensus. Comments from some stakeholders, however, highlighted that this mode of decision making had some drawbacks. These stakeholders reported that, on occasion, risk taking was avoided and consensus was achieved at the expense of diversity in the viewpoints expressed. Difficult social issues tend to be controversial, with community members having many strong points of view, a situation that might not be conducive to consensus decision making. As one stakeholder commented, "We started out great but then started to squelch problems and new opinions and solutions, so a lot left and haven't come back."

CHCI produced benefits for both individuals and groups in terms of creating opportunities for skills to increase and for community members to enhance their abilities to accomplish community work. Stakeholders' reports of the increases in their abilities, due to the planning process, are shown in Table 2.2. At the individual level in particular, many stakeholders said that they had increased their ability to understand community problems, to collaborate productively with others, to develop creative projects to address community problems, and to take a more active leadership role in their community. Those reporting "some" increase or "a great deal" of increase in their areas ranged from 62% to 79%. Stakeholders' perceived ability to personally affect community change also increased; at the end of the planning phase, 52% reported that they were "somewhat more able" to do this, and 11% reported that they were "significantly more able" to do this. At the group level, the large majority of stakeholders believed that they had increased their ability to work effectively with key "power people" in the community (61% reported "some" increase or "a great deal" of increase) and that they had laid a foundation for future work together (63% reported "probably yes" or "definitely yes").

Implementation Phase

In keeping with the CHCI principle to include a broad representation of the community, groups maintained broad and active partnerships with diverse sectors of their communities during the implementation phase. These partnerships varied from formal coalitions and collaborations to informal cooperation and coordination. Although maintaining partnerships is challenging and requires attention and hard work, such partnerships were important to facilitate successful activities.

During the implementation phase, the CHCI projects, on average, undertook six sets of primary activities around different issues. Most of these activities were those that had been originally proposed, but many communities also took on an additional project or two, in part as a response to new opportunities that arose from new partnerships.

Table 2.2   Outcomes of Planning Process: Capacity Building Among Individuals

Capacity Areas and Response Categories	Percentage of Stakeholders
Increase in ability to understand community problems as a result of the planning process $(N = 593)$[a]	
None	7.6
A little	13.7
Some	50.1
A great deal	28.7
Increase in ability to collaborate productively with other community members as a result of the planning process $(N = 594)$[a]	
None	6.4
A little	17.3
Some	52.2
A great deal	24.1
Increase in ability to develop creative projects to address community problems as a result of the planning process $(N = 589)$[a]	
None	13.4
A little	19.4
Some	50.1
A great deal	17.1
Increase in ability to take a more active leadership role in community affairs as a result of the planning process $(N = 590)$[a]	
None	16.9
A little	20.5
Some	46.3
A great deal	16.3
Feel more able to personally effect change in community as a result of the year-long planning process $(N = 1,051)$	
Less able	2.2
No change	35.6
Somewhat more able	51.7
Significantly more able	10.6
Increase in ability to work effectively with key power people in the larger community as a result of the planning process $(N = 343)$[b]	
None	19.0
A little	19.5
Some	47.5
A great deal	14.0
Feel that the planning process built a foundation for future work $(N = 1,057)$	
Definitely no	1.8
Probably no	8.9
Unsure	26.6
Probably yes	41.6
Definitely yes	21.1

a. Asked only during Cycles 2 and 3.
b. Asked only during Cycle 3.

Table 2.3   Primary Implementation Areas Across CHCI Communities

Area	Percentage
Issue focused (61%)	
Illness, wellness	18
Environment	12
Children, youth, and elderly	11
Families	10
Economy	4
Employment	2
Housing	2
Education	2
Structure/Context focused (31%)	
Institutionalize the CHCI process	10
Communication	9
Citizen participation and leadership	6
Community development	6
Fund-raising (8%)	8

NOTE: Total number of implementation areas = 168.

Using the same analysis framework described earlier to classify the KPAs in the communities' visions from the planning phase (issue focused vs. structure/context focused), the primary activities that communities actually undertook during the implementation phase were categorized; Table 2.3 displays the results. The majority of all the communities' primary activities addressed specific issues in the communities such as programs for youth development, with these issue-focused activities comprising 61% of all activities completed. Notably, most of the other activities (31%) focused on community structure/context topics such as fostering citizen participation and increasing leadership ability among citizens (79% of the CHCI communities had at least one structure/content-focused project, and most had two or three such projects). The large majority of CHCI communities, therefore, not only thought about structure/context issues at the time of planning but also acted on these issues during implementation; indeed, the proportion of structure/context focuses, from among the total set of focuses, increased from the planning phase to the implementation phase (from 25% to 31%). Most CHCI communities, therefore, saw the importance of having both issue-focused and structure/context-focused activities to achieve a new vision of health for their communities. Some communities also identified a new category of activity that was important for success: fund-raising (8% of the activities were in this area).

Based on activities and projects actually implemented and completed, a majority of CHCI projects (61%) undertook actions "important to their community," as assessed by independent raters who reviewed the periodic progress reports from all of the communities over the course of the implementation phase. An additional 18% conducted "moderately important" actions. These ranged from issue-focused activities or outcomes, such as the creation of a new family resource center that facilitated family services, to community development-focused outcomes, such as the formation of a civic forum that catalyzed community involvement. Issue-focused actions, however, were more common than community development-focused actions.

By the end of their 2- to 3-year implementation period, a small number of CHCI projects were beginning to show longer term effects of their efforts to change community decision making and governance. At that time, in a few communities (6%), citizens involved with CHCI were influencing community-wide decision making in ways that can have the greatest potential for significant community-level change. These include actions such as participating regularly with important community decision-making bodies (e.g., the county board) and working toward significant policy changes (e.g., in areas such as transportation and land use). At the conclusion of CHCI and of the formal evaluation, therefore, there was some evidence that, at least in a few cases, communities were moving on a new and different path, via more democratic participation of more citizens, toward a healthier future. However, the sustainability of the communities' projects and activities and the institutionalization of changes in community decision making are challenging to maintain. These issues are evaluated in a follow-up study conducted by Larson, Christian, Olson, Hicks, and Sweeney (2002) for The Colorado Trust.

Cross-Initiative

An active, vital coalition of all CHCI projects formed during the planning phase. This informal coalition shared valuable experiences, insights, and support, and it eventually grew into an independent organization, the Colorado Center for Healthy Communities. For several years, this group assisted other individuals and new communities in similar efforts and also provided guidance as the original CHCI communities continued their work. At this point in time, the center no longer exists as a regular organization but has shifted to a virtual organization, with several volunteers providing guidance to those who visit the Web site.

Some of the CHCI communities currently have individualized community-based indicators in place. These indicator sets are as varied as the communities, containing measures of many different key issues, from housing to transportation to economic development. These sets of measures allow the communities to track the progress they are making toward achieving their vision of healthy communities. (See Chapter 3 for a description of this component of CHCI.)

Assessment of the Initiative

The CHCI projects' experiences provide several primary lessons for other communities about to start similar programs or for communities currently involved in healthy cities and communities work.

PLANNING

Achieving meaningful representation of diverse community members requires sensitivity, time, and patience. This applies particularly to minority racial/ethnic members but also to those such as youth and lower income community members. CHCI groups were genuinely interested in reflecting the diversity of their communities, but achieving representativeness was generally not successful in these areas. A more comprehensive and effective way in which to achieve representativeness involves a shift in the CHCI model from *representativeness* to *participation*—genuinely giving diverse citizens a "seat at the table." Success in achieving participation requires early contact with prospective stakeholders, considerable listening and learning, enrollment of these people as collaborators and co-creators of the process, and then adaptation of the model steps and procedures to accommodate everyone's views and ways of doing things.

Consensus decision making has both strengths and weaknesses. At its best, it allows everyone's opinions to be heard, considered, and incorporated into a decision that all can accept. However, the process of reaching consensus can also result in less risk taking and less creative ideas for action. These weaknesses can be ameliorated by condensing the early steps in the planning phase that do not involve much decision making and making more time for the later steps in which consensus plays a large role. This would relieve the pressure for quick decisions (which contributes to easier status quo thinking and less ambitious goals) and would allow more time for stakeholders to explore new ideas and different options for action.

Citizens easily understood and adopted a broad definition of health, involving a social and political view of a healthy community. Communities' definitions included issues well beyond the usual illness focus and extended to aspects of community governance and citizen involvement.

Many individual and group capacities were developed, but other skills and competencies likely to be needed by individuals and groups could be further addressed. These skills include conflict resolution, communication/marketing, and fund-raising.

IMPLEMENTATION

The CHCI process catalyzes action in different areas from those typically addressed by health promotion projects. Many communities undertook issue-focused activities on topics that are rarely considered "health" but, in fact, have significant impacts on whether people are physically and mentally healthy. Examples of issue-focused activities include housing projects for seniors and employment training for community members. In addition, some CHCI communities undertook community process-focused activities on topics that have no direct relationship to improved health but, by changing the way in which communities conduct community business, can empower greater numbers of citizens to become involved in community life and to participate in setting the agenda for community action. An example of a community process-focused activity might include the development of a community forum. Partnerships and collaborations—both individual and organizational—that developed during the planning phase, and that continued during the implementation phase, facilitated the successful implementation of these actions.

There is a tendency for communities' actions to focus more on *issues* than on more general community development *processes*. This is probably due to the fact that actions directed at issues, in contrast to those directed at processes, are easier for most people to understand and undertake and are more likely to produce quick concrete outcomes that may lead to positive effects. Actions directed at processes, such as increased collective community participation, are more unusual and less well understood by most people and tend to produce more diffuse outcomes that take time to result in positive effects. Both issue and process actions are necessary if healthy community processes such as CHCI are to accomplish their goal of empowering citizens to make their communities healthier. Actions directed at process may require extra nurturing, both through examples and models of successful actions from other communities and through special support as the actions unfold. This support could include assistance from and networking with other communities as well as services from facilitators or issue experts.

The desired ultimate objectives of the CHCI process are to create change in community decision making and to improve the health and well-being of citizens. Although some of these changes began to appear in a few CHCI communities, they generally take time and can be difficult to track. To follow these changes over a long period of time, communities need sets of indicators that they can track and measure; these indicators should be based on community-specific definitions of health. In 15 communities, CHCI demonstrated that the creation and implementation of community indicators not only was possible but also provided a way for the communities to track and measure their progress in achieving goals. These results suggest that healthy community processes such as CHCI should include the development of a set of indicators near the beginning of the process to help guide the process and provide a practical way in which to track progress over time. (See Chapter 3 for additional implications.)

Conclusions

CHCI, like the healthy communities model on which it was based, is an ambitious initiative aimed at changing community health by catalyzing and empowering community members and community-based groups to make their communities healthier. Unlike traditional community-*placed* health promotion projects (Baker, 1997), outside experts were not the people who defined the focuses and the activities for the CHCI communities. The idea was that the people who know the community best—the local citizens from many different sectors and perspectives—would define the issues and create the approaches (sometimes with the help of outside experts) that they believed would work best for them. Then they would work to implement their projects and make progress toward a healthier future.

Is this model effective? There are many aspects of the approach that one could question. Do citizens want to have this level of intensive involvement in community-focused work? Can citizens identify health priorities and develop effective projects? Is there a role for experts? Can citizens maintain their involvement over the course of several years? Are there benefits for participants beyond the hope of making their communities healthier? Do communities begin to change as a result of their efforts? Based on the results from the CHCI study, we can provide answers to many of these questions.

Do citizens want intensive involvement in community-focused work? During the planning phase, an average of 50 citizens per community devoted about 1 day per month for nearly 2 years to CHCI work; many of the participants gave even more time. Although some participants at times reported frustration with the lengthy planning period, it is notable that most participants joined the process early, attended most of the meetings, and stayed to the end. Across a variety of Colorado communities, therefore, a sizable number of citizens were intensively involved in community-focused work during the planning phase.

Involvement lessened during the implementation phase. The number of community members involved was less, and those who were involved tended to have more limited involvement than was the case during the planning phase. This may have been less a result of waning citizen interest and more a consequence of a less structured process that was less supportive of citizen involvement as well as a consequence of a hired staff-driven implementation phase, which left less for citizens to do.

Can citizens identify health priorities? The CHCI communities demonstrated that citizens can identify health priorities when health is broadly defined. Although the priorities they identify may be different from those that a health expert might select (e.g., housing as opposed to breast cancer), the process of identifying the priorities engages the citizens in a way that does not occur when a health expert predefines the priorities. Furthermore, this engagement results in more citizen commitment to the eventual programs than normally would occur. However data based and well intentioned, an outside expert's identification of a health agenda is overlaid on a community rather than developed from within the community. This difference, as other researchers have shown (see, e.g., Minkler, 1997), has important implications for subsequent commitment to and ownership of the intervention programs.

Can citizens create innovative programs? The answer to this question is less clear. In the ideal case, CHCI communities were to identify potential project targets (i.e., KPAs) and then invite in experts related to these areas so that they could learn about innovative, cutting-edge programs and models. In practice, CHCI communities did not have the time or the knowledge to do this, although they seemed to be open to this as an option. The fact that outside experts were not used in the CHCI case demonstrates that communities, when left on their own and with little time available at the point where projects are being determined, will turn to local community members for program ideas. Understandably, these people tend to have a more traditional framework and approach. Without expert guidance, communities are not likely to be—and cannot be expected to be—innovative program developers, and the CHCI experience demonstrates this. Within this initiative as implemented, however, the ability of communities to invite in and work with topic-area experts to craft and implement innovative projects was not tested.

Can citizens maintain their involvement over the course of several years? A large number of citizens were involved for the better part of 2 years during the planning phase; this tended not to be the case during the implementation phase. The generally high level of involvement during the planning phase probably resulted from several factors that distinguished the planning and implementation phases. First, the highly structured nature of the planning phase, in contrast to the largely unstructured nature of the implementation phase, gave participants natural tasks and roles. Second, there was regular and intensive involvement of two outside professional facilitators during planning, in contrast to the very limited, sporadic, and problem-focused nature of one facilitator's involvement during the implementation phase. Participants generally gave their planning phase facilitators high marks for their work and mentioned them among the best parts of the planning process; implementation phase facilitators were so rarely involved that most stakeholders were not even aware of them. The planning phase facilitators' regular and intensive involvement explicitly and implicitly signaled to participants that they were on the right path and making progress; this fostered continued participation. During the implementation phase, in contrast, one facilitator would occasionally be involved, usually as a result of a problem or challenge. There was no regular facilitator encouragement, therefore, fostering continued or expanded participation; stakeholders, for the most part, were on their own.

Another difference between the planning and implementation phases that explains different levels of stakeholder involvement relates to the fact that the implementation phase usually involved paid staff who stakeholders viewed as responsible for action, thereby lessening the perceived need for their involvement. During the planning phase, the "staff" were the stakeholders themselves. More stakeholders might have been involved during the implementation phase if there had been a much more structured implementation phase, with activities, exercises, and benchmarks focused on the maintenance and continuation of the stakeholder group and on the refinement, assessment, and tracking of their mission and vision. In addition, if there had been regular facilitation (from either the outside or the inside), this might have nurtured the growth and maturation of the stakeholder group during the latter years of the program.

Are there benefits for participants beyond the hope of making their communities healthier? Stakeholders reported enjoying and learning from the planning meetings. These learnings included some skill development (e.g., how to facilitate meetings) as well as increased knowledge about the community, its assets and challenges, and its people. In addition, stakeholders often met new people with whom they might later work, so there were often personal benefits.

Do communities begin to change as a result of their efforts? The evidence from the CHCI study is limited on this question. In a few cases, communities were beginning to change but, at best, were only at the first stage of such changes. This was true whether the possible improvements were related to particular topics (e.g., transportation) or the process of community decision making. The types of change typically being considered tend to require a long time frame, tend to follow a convoluted path during implementation, and are only part of a larger context with many influences on the community. The CHCI approach, even if very effective, is likely to have been only one contributing factor in explaining community-level changes or the lack of them.

In sum, CHCI demonstrates that a community-based and community-directed approach can provide one way in which to begin the process of promoting health at the community level. Across a diverse set of Colorado communities, large numbers of citizens were centrally involved in defining community health and creating new projects to achieve their visions of what a healthy community could be. The planning process, in particular, empowered the participants and increased their individual capacities to understand and work toward healthy conditions. The CHCI experience clearly demonstrates that large groups of citizens are interested in playing a central role in making their communities healthier and that they have the patience and persistence to work toward a healthy future for their communities. Although the path to achieving their visions of health is a long and challenging one, the CHCI process provides a good start on that path.

Notes

1.   The term "citizen" was used throughout CHCI by the communities, by The Colorado Trust and National Civic League staffs, and by the evaluation team. By this, they meant members of a community or residents of a community. This term is used with the same meaning in this chapter and is interchangeable with "resident," "community member," "stakeholder," and "participant."

2.   More details about the background of the project, as well as about the project model, operation, and participating communities, can be found in Conner et al. (1998).

3.   The consultant funds typically were combined with the other CHCI funds and used for general project operational expenses.

4.   Limited data are presented here. The four primary evaluation reports (Conner et al., 1998; Conner, Tanjasiri, Davidson, et al., 1999; Conner, Tanjasiri, Dempsey, et al., 1999; Conner, Tanjasiri, & Easterling, 1999) contain detailed evaluation data about the results of CHCI.

5.   Stakeholders were able to check more than one choice for the sectors and interests they represented.

References

Baker, Q. E. (1997). *What does community based mean?* Durham, NC: Center for the Advancement of Community Based Public Health.

Conner, R. F., Tanjasiri, S. P., Davidson, M., Dempsey, C., & Robles, G. (1998). *Citizens making their communities healthier: A description of the Colorado Healthy Communities Initiative.* Denver: The Colorado Trust.

Conner, R. F., Tanjasiri, S. P., Davidson, M., Dempsey, C., & Robles, G. (1999). *The first steps toward healthier communities: Outcomes from the planning phase of the Colorado Healthy Communities Initiative.* Denver: The Colorado Trust.

Conner, R. F., Tanjasiri, S. P., Dempsey, C., & Robles, G. (1999). *Working toward healthy communities: Outcomes from the implementation phase of the Colorado Healthy Communities Initiative.* Denver: The Colorado Trust.

Conner, R. F., Tanjasiri, S. P., & Easterling, D. (1999). *Communities tracking their quality of life: An overview of the Community Indicators Project of the Colorado Healthy Communities Initiative.* Denver: The Colorado Trust.

Goodman, R., Speers, M. A., McLeroy, K., Fawcett, S., Kegler, M., Parker, E., Smith, S. R., Sterling, T. D., & Wallerstein, N. (1998). Identifying and defining the dimensions of community capacity to provide a basis for measurement. *Health Education and Behavior, 25,* 258–278.

Larson, C., Christian, A., Olson, L., Hicks, D., & Sweeney, C. (2002). *Colorado Healthy Communities Initiative: Ten years later.* Denver: The Colorado Trust.

Minkler, M. (Ed.). (1997). *Community organizing and community building for health.* New Brunswick, NJ: Rutgers University Press.

Norris, T. (1993). *Colorado healthy communities handbook.* Denver, CO: National Civic League.

World Health Organization. (1995). *WHO Healthy Cities: A programme framework.* Geneva: Author.

3

The Community
Indicators Project

Tracking Health and Quality of Life

Ross F. Conner

Douglas V. Easterling

Sora Park Tanjasiri

James V. Adams-Berger

C hapter 2 presented an overview of the Colorado Healthy Communities Initiative (CHCI) and provided a detailed description of the community-based planning process that served as the point of departure for local stakeholder groups. This chapter focuses on the Community Indicators Project (CIP), which supported roughly half of the CHCI groups in developing a set of *indicators* that could be used to monitor their communities' health and quality of life.

Background

THE POWER OF INDICATORS

One of the simplest, yet most powerful, tools for maintaining and promoting an individual's health is the blood pressure monitor. Knowing a person's blood pressure facilitates the diagnosis of acute illness, chronic disease, and underlying risks to health, which in turn is the first step to taking appropriate remedial action. Depending on the diagnosis, the remedy might involve a short-term intervention (e.g., antibiotics if the patient is plagued with an infection) or a longer term change in lifestyle (e.g., more exercise and less red meat if the person has an elevated risk of cardiovascular disease). Instruments such as thermometers, stethoscopes, and blood assays operate under the same basic logic; measuring a person's health status by any of these means initiates a chain of decision making and action that improves that person's health.

Whereas measuring the health status of an individual can result in significant improvements in *personal* health, measuring the health status of a *community* can promote health on a larger scale. In an effort to measure community-level health, many towns, cities, counties, and states have begun to depend on *community indicators* (Andrews, 1996; Gahin & Paterson, 2001; Redefining Progress, Tyler Norris Associates, & Sustainable Seattle, 1997). Under this approach, measures are found for each of the factors that are important to community health, and then these measures are "observed" and reported at various points in time. For example, a county might rely on indicators such as age-adjusted cancer incidence and immunization rates to assess its physical health along with indicators such as the unemployment rate and median income to assess its economic health. The basic idea behind community indicators is to use a variety of quantitative measures to describe how well the community is doing on critical dimensions. The set of indicators should be broad enough to reflect the entire "system" yet concise enough that the user does not become lost in the details, just as medical *vital signs* (e.g., body temperature, blood pressure, pulse, respiration) provide an efficient overview of a person's physiological functioning. Ideally, indicators are tracked on an ongoing basis and thus provide a means of assessing progress toward a healthy community.

Community indicators act as a tool for health promotion by raising public awareness of what is going well and what is threatening the community's well-being. According to Meadows (1998), "Indicators are a necessary part of the stream of information we use to understand the world, make decisions, and plan our actions" (p. 1). By disseminating indicator data throughout the community (e.g., through newspaper stories, Web sites, or public presentations), local residents, elected officials, businesses, and nonprofit organizations gain a better understanding of the key issues facing the community and can begin to focus their energies and resources in a more concerted way.

COMMUNITY INDICATORS IN PRACTICE

Community indicators are not a recent phenomenon. They have their roots during the early 1800s when social reformers in Philadelphia counted the number of persons in jail awaiting trial as an indicator of the inefficiency and unfairness of the criminal justice system (Cobb & Rixford, 1998). Around 1910, the Russell Sage Foundation provided technical assistance to community groups around the country to support the collection of social indicator data (e.g., education, recreation, public health, crime). These data collection efforts were designed to bring social ills to public attention and to trigger appropriate reform efforts.

> Surveys were conducted under the supervision of citizens' committees, church federations, chambers of commerce, or civic improvement organizations. These groups then relayed the findings of the technical experts to the public who, enlightened by the facts, were expected to mobilize public opinion and press for appropriate reforms. (Smith, 1991, p. 41, quoted in Cobb & Rixford, 1998)

During recent years, more sophisticated versions of community indicators projects have emerged from nonprofit and government agencies throughout the United States and Canada. The Jacksonville Community Council Inc. (JCCI) in Florida developed one of the earliest and longest running indicators projects. Each year since 1985, JCCI has published *Quality of Life in Jacksonville: Indicators for Progress,* an accounting of where the city stands on 82 indicators in areas such as education, the economy, health, natural environment, and government/politics (Besleme, Maser, & Silverstein, 1999; JCCI, 2001). JCCI has succeeded in institutionalizing its indicators project by involving the chamber of commerce and government officials in the production and promotion of the report each year. At the same time, JCCI has developed effective methods for engaging the broader public in the process of responding to the data, including a "citizen-based study process." Over the years, JCCI has served as a leader in innovating new approaches to enhance the impact of community indicators projects on local decision making.

A second pioneering project that serves as a model in the field is *Sustainable Seattle* (AtKisson, 1996). Whereas JCCI uses "quality of life" as its framework for measuring local conditions, this nonprofit organization based in Seattle, Washington, focuses on the somewhat narrower concept of "sustainability," which considers how well a community's ecological, cultural, and human resources are preserved and promoted in the face of population growth and economic expansion. In line with the ethic of "sustainable development," environmental issues play a prominent role in *Sustainable Seattle's* choice of indicators. For example, the report measures how the community performs on dimensions such as the number of wild salmon returning to spawn, the biodiversity of the local plant population, and the degree to which Seattle's streets are "pedestrian-friendly." Since the mid-1990s, community indicators projects such as those in Jacksonville and Seattle have sprouted in cities, counties, regions, and states across the United States. These projects vary greatly in their technical sophistication and formality. At one extreme is the State of Maine's *Measures of Growth,* a high-profile report published each year by the Maine Development Foundation, a nonprofit economic development organization chartered by the legislature. At the other extreme are nascent grassroots efforts that struggle to gain the attention of local officials. To support these projects, organizations such as Redefining Progress (California), Rocky Mountain Institute (Colorado), Urban Quality Communications (Michigan), and Green Mountain Institute (Vermont) have taken a leadership role in developing and disseminating effective models for community indicators projects through listservs, publications, and conferences.

FRAMEWORKS FOR
COMMUNITY INDICATORS PROJECTS

Community indicators projects have used a variety of conceptual frameworks to organize their data collection and to generate recommendations. These include *quality of life, sustainable development, progress, healthy communities, social capital, community report cards, community caring,* and *improving children's lives.* Regardless of the frame of reference, community indicators projects, by definition, measure community well-being along a broad range of dimensions (e.g., economic well-being, the natural environment, arts and culture, recreation, and civic participation).

Although all community indicators projects are *inclusive* in the sense that they include a variety of indicators, projects vary in terms of how many people are included in the process of choosing the indicators. In particular, community indicators projects tend to fall into one of two distinct categories: (a) *advocacy* projects that use indicators to promote a particular position or perspective and (b) *collective definition* projects that try to develop a set of indicators that will reflect the community's collective sense of health or quality of life.

Under the *advocacy* model, indicators serve as a tool for advancing a particular organization's agenda, be it economic development, public health, environmental preservation, or self-promotion. The basic idea is for the organization to find the "best" indicators that represent the organization's own objectives or vision for the community. The lead organization might be a chamber of commerce, an environmental advocacy group, the local health department, or a university. Once the organization decides how to measure progress toward its own vision of a "good society," it collects the data, creates a report, and then brings the findings to key "stakeholders" or "decision makers"—the various individuals, agencies, institutions, and firms whose actions and decisions influence the life of the community. The objective is to convince the key stakeholders that the selected indicators provide the right criteria to guide policymaking and budgeting within the government sector as well as the programming and spending decisions made by nonprofit organizations, funders, businesses, economic development agencies, health departments, and others.

In contrast, *collective definition* indicators projects are much more broad based in engaging local citizens in the selection of indicators and the definition of what should be measured. Whereas advocacy projects start with a political agenda that determines how quality of life will be measured, this second type of indicator project starts with a cross section of the public whose members develop a consensus definition of what "quality of life" means within their community. Indicators are not selected until this more basic question has been resolved in a way that satisfies the various sectors that make up the community. Thus, rather than using indicators to make a case for one particular organization's point of view, these projects use indicators to reach a clearer understanding of the community's deeper underlying values in measurable terms. In other words, the community indicators project serves as a tool for collective self-discovery. According to Meadows (1993), "The idea of citizens choosing their indicators is something new under the sun—something intensely democratic" (p. 24).

BRINGING COMMUNITY INDICATORS TO COLORADO

The Colorado Trust's CIP was grounded in the second of these two philosophical frameworks. Under CIP, 15 communities were funded to initiate a process to identify locally relevant indicators of health and quality of life. Each community was encouraged to define "health" and "quality of life" according to its own unique set of values. This approach was based on the assumption that only through an in-depth, locally driven process of indicator selection would the measurement task become valid and meaningful and, thus, have any substantive impact on local decision making. CIP qualifies as an instance of *community-based* health promotion because (a) each project was managed by a local organization (e.g., municipal government, university, nonprofit) and (b) local residents and organizations decided which indicators would be included in their report.[1]

Even though CIP is community based, one might still question whether this is a tool for *health promotion* because community indicators typically measure conditions beyond physical illness and wellness. We would argue that it is vital to pay attention to a broad range of quality of life measures if one is interested in promoting health. This view builds on the broad conception of *health* that the World Health Organization has fostered over the past few decades (World Health Organization, 1946, 1986). In measuring how healthy we are at any given time, we look not only at our physiological functioning but also at our emotional, mental, and spiritual balance. Likewise, a healthy *community* is now regarded as a place where the residents are healthy (physically, emotionally, mentally, and spiritually) and where the various systems that define community life (economic, environmental, cultural, political, and social) are operating to support local residents (World Health Organization, 1986). Even when considering "health" from its narrowest definition, it is now clear that "social determinants" such as poverty and social support play a major role in determining how long people live and how free from disease and injury their lives are (Wilkinson & Marmot, 1998).

This chapter provides an overview of the structure of CIP and some of the preliminary results and lessons that have emerged over the first 5 years of the project. It includes a detailed case description of one of the projects to illustrate how the process worked in practice.

The Community Indicators Project

ORIGINS

The Colorado Trust created the Community Indicators Project as an extension of CHCI (described in Chapter 2). Launched in 1992, CHCI supported broad-based coalitions in 28 Colorado communities in finding effective, locally relevant strategies to improve "health," broadly defined. Under CHCI, a group of representative stakeholders was convened in each community to explore the issues, threats, trends, and opportunities that influenced the health and quality of life of local residents. The stakeholder group then developed an action agenda of projects designed to address the key "leverage points" that emerged during the 15-month planning process.[2]

As part of the CHCI planning model, each community developed a *Community Health Profile,* a compilation of community-specific data that allowed the planning group to recognize and understand trends in various health and quality of life issues. These profiles typically relied on existing data reports (e.g., from the local health department, the criminal justice system, the state demographer, or various economic agencies) that the planning group could access in short order. To varying degrees, the data in these Community Health Profiles informed the planning group's choice of issues to address through its action projects. In addition, some communities published summaries of the data to help other local organizations (e.g., government agencies, nonprofit organizations) make more informed decisions and prepare more competitive grant proposals.

CIP was designed to provide a means for CHCI-funded communities to extend the work they had performed in developing their Community Health Profiles. Whereas the profile was a one-time project intended to inform a strategic plan, CIP was designed to support the development of an ongoing "index" that would allow CHCI communities to assess how well they were progressing toward their respective visions of a healthy community.[3]

The addition of a community indicators element to CHCI was in keeping with the "healthy communities" philosophy, which emphasizes citizen-driven processes for defining health and setting health promotion priorities (Ashton, 1992; Hancock & Duhl, 1986; Kickbusch, 1989). Throughout the country, a number of healthy communities projects have adopted social indicators following their planning processes to track progress on their action plans (Besleme & Mullin, 1997; Gross & Straussman, 1974; Innes, 1990; Land, 1992).

As The Colorado Trust began to explore the possibility of creating a "mini-initiative" to support the development of community indicators among CHCI projects, many of the grantees expressed a strong interest in the idea. One CHCI grantee, Healthy Mountain Communities, had already begun the process of creating an indicators report, which piqued the interest of a few other CHCI communities. The Colorado Healthy Communities Council (a network formed by the CHCI grantees in 1995 as a means of sharing ideas and reducing isolation) provided an explicit endorsement of this new direction by highlighting community indicators at its 1995 and 1996 annual conferences.

SELECTION OF GRANTEES

CIP was launched in the fall of 1995 with the release of a request for proposals (RFP) to those CHCI coalitions that had completed their planning process. Of the 19 eligible communities, 12 submitted proposals and 8 were selected for funding. These 8 communities began developing community indicators in January 1996. In the fall of that year, The Colorado Trust issued a second RFP to the remaining CHCI communities and awarded CIP grants to 7 sites. Thus, 15 of the 28 CHCI communities were funded under CIP.

The geographic boundaries of the 15 participating communities are shown in the map in Figure 3.1. The CIP communities were a mix of urban, rural, and frontier localities. Of the 15 communities, 3 were incorporated cities in the Denver metro area (Aurora, Commerce City, and Lakewood), 7 were single-county areas (Boulder, Chaffee, Custer, Mesa, Montezuma, Pueblo, and Weld), and 5 were multicounty regions (Healthy Mountain Communities, Operation Healthy Communities [OHC], San Luis Valley, Uncompahgre, and Yampa Valley). The largest community is the six-county San Luis Valley, which extends over 8,143 square miles between the San Juan and Sangre de Cristo mountains (slightly less than the size of New Hampshire). The 15 communities varied greatly in population size, from 2,700 to 249,000, with a median of 42,000 residents.

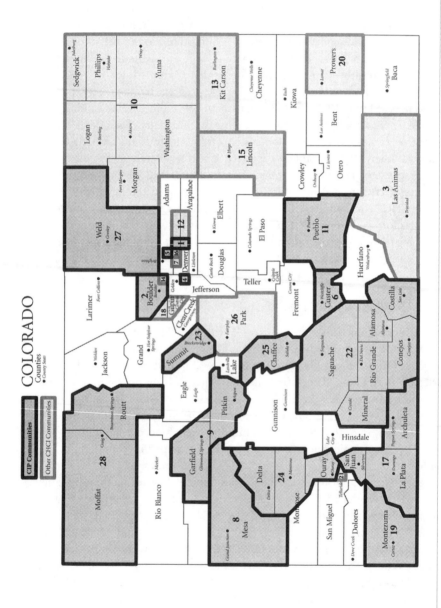

Figure 3.1   Map of Communities That Participated in CIP

Key to the Healthy Communities

*1. The Aurora Project (*City of Aurora*)
*2. Boulder County Healthy Communities Initiative
3. CHANCE (*Las Animas County*) *now hosted by Fisher's Peak YMCA*
*4. Citizens for Lakewood's Future (*City of Lakewood*)
*5. Commerce City: Mission Possible!
*6. Custer 2020 (*Custer County*)
7. Globeville Community Connection (*North Denver neighborhood*)
*8. Healthy Community 2000 (*Mesa County*) *now known as Mesa County Healthy Community Civic Forum*
*9. Healthy Mountain Communities (*Garfield, Pitkin and western Eagle counties*)
10. Healthy Plains Initiative (*Logan, Morgan, Phillips, Sedgwick, Washington and Yuma counties*)
*11. Healthy Pueblo 2000 (*Pueblo County*) *now known as Healthy Pueblo Communities 2010*
12. High Five Plains Vision for 2015 (*I-70 Corridor—includes the towns of Bennett, Byers, Deer Trail, Strasburg and Watkins*)
13. Kit Carson County Healthy Communities Initiative (*Kit Carson County*) *now hosted by Healthy Living System, Inc.*
14. Lafayette Healthy Communities (*City of Lafayette*)
15. Linc-Up (*Lincoln County*)
16. Neighbors Connecting for a Healthy Future (*Northeast Denver—City Park, City Park West, Cole, Five Points, North Capitol hill and Whittier neighborhoods*) *implementation project is now called Center for Self Help & Development*
*17. Operation Healthy Communities (*Archuleta, La Plata and San Juan counties*)
18. Peak to Peak Healthy Communities Project (*Gilpin County & the Nederland mountain area*)
*19. The Pinon Project (*Montezuma County, including the Ute Mountain Ute Tribe*)
20. Prowers' Progress to a Healthy Future (*Prowers County*)
21. REACH (*Telluride Region*)
*22. San Luis Valley Community Connections (*Alamosa, Conejos, Costilla, Mineral, Rio Grande and Saguache counties*)
*23. Shaping Our Summit (*Summit County*)
*24. Uncompahgre Healthy Communities Project (*Delta, Ouray & eastern Montrose counties & the Somerset area of Gunnison County*)
*25. Valley Visions (*Chaffee County*)
26. Vision 2020 (*Park County*)
*27. Vision Together (*Weld County*) *now known as Weld Citizen Action Network*
*28. Yampa Valley Partners (*Moffat and Routt counties*)

---

*Communities funded under CIP.
**Additional community that carried out an indicator project.

SUPPORT TO GRANTEES

Each of the 15 CHCI organizations funded under CIP was granted up to $48,000 over a 2-year period. These funds were used to pay for a part-time staff person and other project expenses (e.g., travel, data management, preparation of reports). In addition, The Colorado Trust provided grantees with technical assistance from OMNI Institute of Denver and sponsored three networking conferences per year.

At the beginning of CIP, technical assistance was delivered according to a fairly traditional, expert-oriented model. Researchers from OMNI visited each site and provided advice on issues related to the selection of valid and reliable indicators, data management, reporting, and community involvement. After the first year of the project, however, the limitations of the "traveling consultant" model became apparent. The CIP project directors expressed a desire to set their own learning agenda and to support one another in group settings. Thus, the technical assistance model shifted to an approach that relied primarily on workshops in which grantees could share their experiences with one another and where outside speakers could suggest new approaches and perspectives for addressing the myriad challenges associated with developing and using community indicators.[4]

THE ORIGINAL CIP MODEL

CIP was designed to help CHCI-funded coalitions develop relevant, valid indicators reports that would serve as a catalyst to action. More specifically, The Colorado Trust articulated the following two goals in the RFP for CIP:

1. Each funded community will establish a system for measuring, on a regular basis, local health and quality of life.

2. CIP will increase the research skills of individuals doing indicator work in Colorado and will promote more effective practices for the development of indicators.

Figure 3.2 lays out the more specific objectives that The Colorado Trust communicated to grantees.

The local project director was expected to take the lead in developing each community's indicator project by facilitating the indicator selection process, finding data sources, compiling and analyzing the data, and producing the report. At the same time, projects were expected to involve the larger community in a substantive way. CIP was envisioned primarily as a community development project—one where local residents would ask and answer critical

GOAL I: The community will establish a system for measuring, on a regular basis, local health and quality of life.

OBJECTIVE 1: The project will verify and/or refine its vision of a healthy community.

OBJECTIVE 2: Relying on the vision and broad-based community input, the project will identify a set of critical dimensions of health and quality of life that are meaningful to local residents.

OBJECTIVE 3: Again using input from community representatives, the project will identify a set of valid and reliable indicators that measure the agreed-to dimensions. Some of these indicators will rely on existing data sets (e.g., vital statistics), whereas others will involve new data collection.

OBJECTIVE 4: The project will obtain current and historical data showing how the community stands on each indicator. Where appropriate, data will be compiled for significant subunits of the community (e.g., each county within a multicounty community).

OBJECTIVE 5: By the end of the first year, the project will publish a readable report summarizing the indicator data. The indicator report will be widely distributed throughout the community and will be publicized by local media.

OBJECTIVE 6: During the second year, the project will solicit community response to the report and develop a system for improving and sustaining its report.

OBJECTIVE 7: By the end of the second year, the community will commit the resources to continue the preparation and publication of community indicator reports on a regular basis.

GOAL II: CIP will increase the research skills of individuals doing indicator work in Colorado and will promote more effective practices for the development of indicators.

OBJECTIVE 8: The project director will increase his or her skills in the areas of research design, data collection, data analysis, and presentation.

OBJECTIVE 9: The project director will share with other project directors the lessons he or she learns in developing indicator reports.

OBJECTIVE 10: Researchers residing in the funded community will form networks that promote the sharing of data and expertise.

Figure 3.2   CIP Goals and Objectives

questions about the nature of "health" and then take collective and individual actions to address the major issues uncovered by the measurement task.

In addition to the objectives listed in Figure 3.2, CIP was defined by a "recommended" model for selecting indicators. In particular, the CIP steering committee (composed of representatives from The Colorado Trust, OMNI Institute, and the University of California, Irvine, research team) developed a conceptual framework to guide CIP grantees through the process of developing their first indicators reports. This relatively linear process (depicted in Figure 3.3) consisted of six steps: (1) grounding the process with a local vision, (2) identifying broad domains to organize the indicators, (3) deciding on the key dimensions, (4) selecting the indicators, (5) collecting the data, and (6) creating the report. Each step is described in what follows.

1. *Ground the process with a local vision.* Under this first step, the local working group develops a vision statement that articulates what it means for the community to be "healthy." Because each CIP grantee had completed the CHCI planning process, each already had a vision statement. Thus, the grantee's first step was to reassess that vision statement, revise it as necessary, and incorporate any other vision statements that might have emerged from other community-based planning efforts related to health and quality of life. At the end of this step, the working group would have a common framework for answering the following question: What issues do we need to be sure to include if we are to measure the "health" of our community?

2. *Identify broad domains to organize the indicators.* From the vision statement, the working group determines which "domains" are contained in the vision. Domains are general areas of focus such as education, transportation, environment, and health. As the project moves to the task of selecting specific indicators, subcommittees might be formed to focus on the different domains.

3. *Decide on the key dimensions.* Whereas domains serve as broad categories for organizing the selection of indicators, "dimensions" are the more specific aspects of quality of life that the project chooses to measure. For example, within the domain of education, a community might decide that it really cares about three particular aspects: the extent to which students graduate from high school, the degree to which students develop reading and analytic skills, and the level of resources provided to the schools (e.g., financial support, teacher/student ratios). Each of these issues would be a dimension. The challenge is to find the "right" dimensions—those that correspond to the community's underlying value system.

4. *Select the indicators.* The articulation of dimensions essentially defines the measurement task. In particular, the basic goal of a community indicators

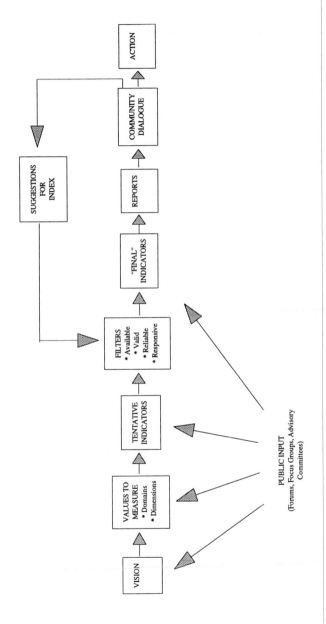

Figure 3.3 The CIP Framework for Developing Community Indicators (initial)

55

project is to find measures that capture the dimensions that local residents regard as central to quality of life.

To continue the preceding example, if during Step 3 the working group determined that the degree to which students develop reading skills is a key dimension, it might choose to include indicators such as the proportion of fourth-grade and eighth-grade students scoring at least "proficient" on a standardized reading test.

In deciding which indicators to include, the working group needs to explore various data sources to determine what is available and then to assess how well the candidate indicators actually reflect the meaning of the various dimensions. This assessment task includes considerations such as the availability of data over time, the reliability and validity of the indicator, whether or not the indicator can be understood by the general public, and whether or not the indicator can be influenced by local actions and decisions. CIP grantees were presented with the checklist of criteria in Table 3.1 to guide the indicator selection process. These criteria were developed by OMNI based on the recommendations of David Swain from the Jacksonville project.

The CIP steering committee encouraged communities to find creative indicators that would accurately capture the fundamental values of local residents rather than compiling statistics solely on the basis of availability or convenience. In addition, CIP promoted the use of "positive" indicators of a community's assets (Kretzmann & McKnight, 1993) rather than focusing solely on problems, deficits, and pathologies.

By positioning the identification of dimensions step before the indicators selection step, CIP grantees were encouraged to ground their indicators in community values. Previous experience has shown that community indicators projects have a tendency to begin by brainstorming specific indicators, which leads to an indicator set that reflects primarily the knowledge and preferences of the people around the table. In contrast, the approach in Figure 3.3 requires the working group to be clear on what it wants to measure before even considering the question of specific indicators.

5. *Collect the data.* Once the indicators are defined, the CIP project director goes to the various data sources (e.g., publications, Web sites), identifies the relevant data, and extracts the data for the project's database. Working group members are involved in this process to the extent that they have "special" access to a particular data source. Most indicators are created by accessing existing data sets. In a few select cases, a project may choose to conduct a survey or use some other data collection method to create an indicator.

6. *Create the report.* Finally, the CIP project director, usually with the help of relevant community members and the advice of the working group, prepares

Table 3.1   Criteria for Selecting Indicators

Issue	Description
Reliability	Is there a consistent way in which to measure the indicator over time? Is there support for continued measurement of the indicator well into the future?
Validity	Is there evidence that the indicator provides meaningful information about the chosen dimension? Will a change in the indicator reflect a change in the dimension? Does an indicator need to be interpreted in relation to other indicators in order to make a judgment about the dimension?
Sensitivity to change	Does the indicator respond quickly and noticeably to real changes? Is the indicator updated frequently enough to demonstrate this change? At what geographic level will the indicator demonstrate change?
Accessibility	Is the indicator available? Is the indicator at the needed geographic level and in the right format—disk, CD-ROM, tape? Is the indicator affordable?
Policy relevance[a]	Does the indicator have relevance for public policy decisions? Can the community do anything that would lead to improvements in the indicator?
Understandability[a]	Is the indicator easily interpreted by the general public?
Political considerations	Is the indicator likely to be controversial for stakeholders or identifiable segments of the community?
Comprehensiveness	Will the indicators, taken as a whole, provide a full picture of the vision statement? If the community makes progress toward the vision, will this show up in more than one indicator?
No redundancy	Do all of the indicators make a unique contribution?
Cost-effectiveness	Do community priorities correspond to where money is being spent on indicators? If primary data collection is being conducted, is the sample size efficient? Can additional information be gathered in the survey with no added cost?
Standardization	Is the set of indicators similar to those used in other countries, states, and the like such that comparisons could be made?

a. Adapted from *Quality Indicators for Progress, A Guide to Community Quality-of-Life Assessments*, a community indicators replication kit developed by the Jacksonville Community Council Inc.

the indicators report in a user-friendly format (with compelling graphics and readable text). The report is then released and actively disseminated in the community.

The CIP steering committee developed this "model process" with the intent of maximizing the visibility and relevance of each grantee's indicators report. In particular, the steering committee believed that if a group followed these steps and engaged key sectors of the community throughout the process, the resulting report would be more likely to have an impact on local decision making and behavior. The recommended approach to selecting indicators (i.e., bringing together a representative group of residents and officials to translate the community's vision into measurable dimensions) was designed to heighten local interest and buy-in. Ideally, this increased attention would, in turn, lead to more responsive informed actions on the part of local elected officials, government agencies, nonprofit organizations, employers, and residents. An example of such an action would be a change in the allocation of local resources (e.g., city and county tax revenues, organizational/agency budgets) to address needs identified through the indicators process.

The Development of Indicators in Colorado Communities

OHC CASE STUDY

In general terms, the model process described previously guided each CIP grantee. For example, the projects were consistent in terms of relying on a vision statement, hiring a project director, creating a working group, and involving the larger community through public forums. At the same time, each CIP-funded community pursued its own unique approach to creating an indicators report under the leadership of the local project director.

To provide a more concrete sense of what the process of developing an indicators report actually involved, this section describes the actual experience of one particular grantee: Operation Healthy Communities.[5] Figure 3.4 shows a sample page from the OHC indicators report. Although this case is unique, it provides a representative illustration of how the various communities adapted the CIP framework to fit their own cultures, histories, and personalities.

Context

OHC is a nonprofit organization in Durango, Colorado, that was created during the implementation phase of CHCI, the larger initiative within which

STRONG, COHESIVE COMMUNITIES

Definition

A significant aspect of the quality and well being of a healthy community is social cohesion and public involvement. Communities gain their strength from an active participation of citizens, from safe neighborhoods, and an open dialogue between community members and government leaders.

Value	Indicators & Measures		Archuleta	Dolores	La Plata	San Juan
Involved Citizens	% registered voters participating in off-year election	1990	60.22%	70.62%	84.00%	70.34%
		1994	56.85%	69.05%	62.58%	54.34%
Open Dialogue between Citizens and Governments **	# of times last year you attended a meeting on a community issue	0	13.64%	*	29.27%	*
		1-3	28.40%		36.75%	
		4-6	18.18%		8.70%	
		7-9	9.10%		4.49%	
		10 or more	30.68%		20.73%	
Strong Neighborhoods **	Do you feel safe walking in your neighborhood at night?	yes	96.6%	*	91.8%	*
		no	3.4%		8.82%	
	Do you feel comfortable asking for or giving something to a neighbor?	yes	93.1%	*	90.98%	*
		no	6.9%		9.02%	

* no data available   ** Information from 1996 United Way survey

Interpretation

A general sense of safety is present within neighborhoods. The measurement of voter participation in all years is close to the state and national average of 72% except in Archuleta County. There was, however, significant decline in the percent of voter participation from 1990 to 1994 in La Plata County. While there is no benchmark for degree of attendance at community meetings, among those surveyed by United Way, over 70% attended at least one meeting in the last year; however, 30% have had no involvement.

Linkages

Continued citizen involvement and open dialogue can serve to overcome the divisions that exist in our communities. As our communities change and grow, it is even more significant that we can concentrate on building strong and cohesive places to live with creative, cooperative problem solving.

Current Activities/Future Suggestions

The development of collaborative efforts or leadership training have occurred with such organizations as Leadership La Plata, Archuleta 2000, OHC's Common Ground Coalition, the South Durango Neighborhood Association, and other neighborhood associations. Collaboration between municipal and county governments may continue to need attention. The work of such groups as the League of Women Voters should also be strengthened and sustained.

> *"...it is only in community that we can be citizens. It is only in community that we can find care. It is only in community that we can hear people singing."*
>
> — John McKnight,
> *The Careless Society: Community and Its Counterfeits*, 1995, p. 172.

Figure 3.4   Sample Page From the OHC Indicators Report

Source: Operation Healthy Communities, 1997. Reprinted by permission.

CIP was developed. OHC serves three counties (Archuleta, La Plata, and San Juan) covering 3,428 square miles in the southwestern portion of the state. This region of high desert and snowcapped mountains includes one city (Durango), four incorporated towns, many small unincorporated towns, five school districts, and the Southern Ute Nation. At the outset of CIP, the area had approximately 38,000 people, consisting mainly of whites but also a significant population of Hispanics and Native Americans. The local economy was historically based on extractive industries (mining, logging, oil, and gas), but tourism had begun to become the dominant sector. Among local residents and elected officials, the dominant issues of concern were population growth (approximately 4% per year), escalating real estate prices, and the need to diversify the economy.

Getting Started

As soon as The Colorado Trust announced the CIP funding opportunity in the fall of 1995, key players within OHC mobilized to lay the groundwork for a community indicators project and to develop a competitive proposal. Marsha Porter-Norton, the director of OHC, and Sam Burns, a professor of sociology at Fort Lewis College who was deeply involved in the CHCI planning process, took the lead in building local buy-in from the public, nonprofit, business, education, and government sectors. They also developed a plan wherein the community indicators project would build on a number of existing research and community development efforts (e.g., the San Juan National Forest's comprehensive planning process, the Region 9 Economic Development District's analysis of employment growth by sector).

After being notified that it had been awarded a CIP grant, OHC hired Lynn Shine, the mayor of Durango, to serve as the project coordinator. Shortly thereafter, OHC convened an "Indicators Council" to represent the various sectors, communities, and interests that make up the three-county region. Participants were selected to represent a particular focus or interest (e.g., education) but also were encouraged to take a broad, area-wide perspective. A conscious effort was made to include traditionally unrepresented perspectives such as those of people with disabilities, the Southern Ute Tribe, and other racial/ethnic groups.

Deciding What Aspects of Quality of Life Need to Be Measured

The first step to developing indicators was to create a local point of reference for measuring quality of life. To do this, the Indicators Council reviewed five different vision statements that had been created by different planning and visioning groups over the previous 5 years. From these vision statements, the council identified the key underlying values and grouped them into four broad categories:

- *Human Services:* Health care, affordable housing, schools, and other human services

- *Quality of Life:* Environment, cultural heritage, community, recreation, and recycling

- *Economy–Transportation–Communication:* Combined into one category, with economy focused on enterprise zones, sustainable agriculture, and a healthy and environment-friendly economy; transportation focused on high-quality air service and safe roads; and communications focused on high-quality telecommunications

- *Family Life:* Healthy families and safe families

These categories are equivalent to the "domain" level in the CIP model, although OHC did not explicitly use the "domain/dimension" terminology.

Selecting Indicators

After agreeing on the four categories of values, the Indicators Council broke into subgroups to find indicators for each one. Each subgroup was instructed to select indicators based on the criteria of: validity, availability and timeliness, stability and reliability, understandability, responsiveness, policy relevance, and representativeness (see Table 3.1). To varying degrees, these criteria informed the brainstorming process that each subgroup undertook to develop possible indicators. During this process, the members began to grapple with their different expectations for indicators, disagreeing on issues such as whether it was more appropriate to use rates or raw counts.

After each subgroup identified a set of indicators to cover its focus area, the full Indicators Council met to combine the separate lists. At this point in the process, the master list consisted of about 125 indicators. To pare down this list, each subgroup reconvened to look for indicators that could be cut. This task was only marginally successful, however, because participants were reluctant to "give up" their preferred indicators. Moreover, new participants joined the process at this point and advocated for additional indicators. After prolonged discussion, the full committee recommended that data be collected on 96 different indicators.

Collecting Data and Revisiting the Indicators List

With the list of preferred indicators in hand, the project coordinator began the task of trying to collect data for each one. Her goal was to find county-level data that went back in time over a period of several years.[6] Some of the desired data were readily available from agency records, statistical publications, and Web sites, but other searches were much more protracted. In some cases, members of the Indicators Council had been confident that a particular indicator existed, but an extended search by the project coordinator proved this to be wishful thinking.

The search for *water quality* data provides a cautionary tale about the availability of valid, reliable, useful indicators. One of the proposed indicators was the *surface water quality* of the region's rivers, but the necessary tests had been performed on only one of the eight river basins in the region. For another indicator, *quality of groundwater*, the project coordinator looked to the well water tests performed by the county health departments. These tests, however, measured contamination resulting from faulty well seals as much as they measured actual chemical contamination of the aquifer. Likewise, the water quality data reported by the U.S. Geological Survey and the Environmental Protection Agency proved to be so complex, technical, and detailed that a special consultant would have had to be hired to interpret them, and even then the data would probably not have produced a meaningful water quality index.

As with all of the CIP projects that covered multicounty regions, OHC ran into difficulty with different jurisdictions using different methods or definitions to collect their data (i.e., a lack of reliability in measurement). For example, in counting attendance at local "arts events," the project coordinator found that different communities employed different criteria to determine what constituted an arts event. Moreover, each community was quite attached to its own definition and unwilling to adopt a standardized version that would promote cross-community measurement and comparison.

The project coordinator's task was even more complicated in cases where the Indicators Council had proposed that new data be collected. For example, the council suggested a survey of mobile home parks to collect data that could be used to create an indicator of *mobile home rental costs*. The project coordinator contacted approximately 30 mobile home parks across the four counties, but many of the owners were suspicious, thinking that competitors were calling to get rate information. The owners were reluctant to return phone calls, much less to provide data.

When problems such as this arose, attempts were made to substitute more valid or accessible indicators. Even so, many of the 96 proposed indicators were removed from the list due to problems with availability, reliability, and/or validity. Thus, the hunt for data included a "funneling down" step. At the same time, new indicators were added to the list. In some cases, a new indicator was added because the working group recognized that it would take more than one indicator to fully capture the underlying value. In other cases, however, a new indicator made its way onto the list due to strong advocacy by key members of the Indicators Council. In the end, data were collected on 99 indicators covering the four categories of values (human services, quality of life, economy–transportation–communication, and family life).

Writing the Report

The Indicators Council determined the format for the report and then created a *writing committee* to fill in the required sections for each category of indicators. As draft sections were prepared, the project coordinator circulated them for review to other key individuals, some of whom had not previously been involved with the project. For example, the section on education indicators was shared with school representatives, whereas the affordable housing indicators were shared with realtors, government officials, and interested citizens. These reviewers were asked to comment on the accuracy of the data and its believability. In several cases, this review process led to the refinement or deletion of an indicator, but always on technical grounds rather than political grounds. At the end of the review process, the comments were incorporated into the document and the final report was assembled, formatted, and published.

The Report

The final report, 59 pages long, is titled *Pathways to Healthier Communities: Archuleta, Dolores, La Plata, and San Juan Counties* (OHC, 1997). In addition to the actual indicator data, the report introduces each indicator topic, with definitions and a vision statement, and presents some implications of the data (i.e., interpretation, linkages with other community issues, current activities related to the issue, and suggestions for future action).

The report is formatted according to a "tree" of values and indicators. The largest branches are the four categories of human services, quality of life, economy–transportation–communications, and family life. Each category has a number of more specific dimensions, and each dimension has a number of even more specific subdimensions (i.e., the smallest branches). Indicators enter into the scheme as measures of the subdimensions (or "leaves" at the end of the branches).

To illustrate this format, consider the category of quality of life. This section of the report begins with a statement of the community's values related to quality of life:

We envision strong, cohesive communities where involved citizens of all ethnic backgrounds work together to preserve our small-town, rural lifestyle, promote stewardship of the land, preserve open space, and value clean air. We envision communities where people have a high regard for their neighbors, have a strong sense of place and attachment to the land, and have a commitment to sustaining a community-oriented way of life. We envision communities that establish an open dialogue between leaders and citizens and where volunteerism is strongly valued. Our communities provide ample opportunities to share cultural heritage, enjoy the arts, and participate in a variety of recreational and cultural events. (OHC, 1997, p. 8)

Following a page of photographs related to quality of life, the report presents four dimensions that underlie this topic: *strong cohesive communities, recreation, healthy environment,* and *cultural heritage.* Each of these dimensions has multiple subdimensions. The dimension of strong cohesive communities is defined in terms of the subdimensions *involved citizens, open dialogue between citizens and government,* and *strong neighborhoods.* The specific indicators for these three subdimensions are shown in Figure 3.4 along with the actual data. Some of the indicators are measured at only a single point in time, whereas others include historical data with measurements at earlier points in time.

With the "tree–branches–leaves" format, the report ties the specific indicator data back to a comprehensive taxonomy of community values. This was designed to provide a "big picture" wherein everyone in the community could find indicators of direct interest while at the same time seeing the strong interconnections among all of the community's issues. Most of the other CIP projects adopted a similar organizing scheme.

OHC published approximately 500 copies of the final report. These were distributed for a nominal fee to local residents and elected officials. Individuals living outside the area who requested the report were charged more so as to generate a small profit. The indicator data were also presented to the community in public forums and through the local newspaper. Because of the broad-based process that OHC had used to review the draft report, many community members were primed for the release of the report.

THE CIP PROCESS ACROSS COMMUNITIES

The experience of OHC provides a concrete example of how an indicators report was produced under CIP. Although the OHC case is *representative* of the process that CIP grantees underwent, each project had its own nuances. This section describes some of the key overarching results from the different projects as they developed their first indicators reports.

In terms of staffing, the CIP grants were not large enough to support a full-time position, so project directors typically worked either as a part-time employee of the local CHCI project or as a contracted consultant. In a few cases, the director of the CHCI organization served as the CIP project director as well. Despite the fact that many of the CIP communities were rural and semi-isolated, each project succeeded in hiring a local resident as its project director. Of the 15 projects, 4 hired directors affiliated with a local college or university; the remainder recruited individuals with backgrounds in regional planning, social services, market research, and/or community development.

The six-step model developed by the CIP steering committee (Figure 3.3) served as a starting point for the local projects but was adapted in various ways to fit the local contexts. In all cases, the selection of indicators was guided by significant community input. Some projects relied heavily on advisory committees made up of both experts in research/measurement and individuals with expertise in the different aspects of quality of life that the indicators seek to capture (e.g., physical health, environment, culture, spirituality, civic participation, economy, housing). Forums and focus groups also served as important mechanisms for incorporating broader community perspectives in many of the projects. In each project, the project director attempted to balance the need to be inclusive (i.e., to reflect the diversity of interests that are represented in the process) with the need to be practical (i.e., to create a set of indicators that is relatively parsimonious and leads to a feasible measurement task). The project director was also responsible for ensuring that the issues of reliability and validity were adequately incorporated into the choice of indicators.

Although the specific process varied across sites, all CIP projects used the vision statement created during the CHCI planning phase as the first step in identifying the "right" indicators. In a few cases, the working group incorporated additional vision statements that had emerged from non-CHCI planning efforts that had taken place in the community. In reviewing the various vision statements, the working group often found that much of the language was too vague to suggest a specific indicator. On the other hand, as the working group struggled with the question of how to measure its vision, the group members sometimes fleshed out their vision statement in more concrete terms.

In moving from vision to indicators, advisory committees typically generated a long list of potential indicators—in some communities, well over 100. The winnowing down and selection processes were guided by two complementary, although potentially competing, considerations. First, diverse representatives from the community needed to help select the most important dimensions within each domain. Second, in selecting specific indicators to reflect these dimensions, participants also had to take into account methodological issues such as reliability and validity as well as the potential for indicators to have an impact on policy decisions (see Table 3.1).

By and large, each CIP site created an indicator set with great breadth. The most common "domains" included economy, health, education, environment, employment, housing, recreation, community participation, crime and violence, poverty, arts and culture, and birth outcomes. Less frequent domains included agriculture, telecommunications, and spirituality.[7] In keeping with the emphasis on a *community-driven* indicator selection process, each CIP community came up with its own unique set of indicators. Although the sites overlapped to some degree in terms of the dimensions they were trying to measure (e.g., immunization levels, amount of "open space," air quality, volunteerism, proportion of families earning a livable wage), they tended to adopt idiosyncratic indicators to tap into those dimensions. During networking meetings, the project directors from the different CIP sites discussed the benefits of using common measures but opted to rely on the recommendations that emerged from their own locally driven process.

A project typically took between 14 and 24 months to produce its first indicators report. The most time-consuming aspects of the project included hiring staff, becoming oriented to the concepts and methods underlying community indicators, convening committees, deliberating on the choice of indicators, finding data, analyzing the data, and formatting and publishing the reports. The strong emphasis on community involvement, combined with the formative nature of the work (the CIP projects were designing and refining their approach as they went), added significantly to the time that was required to produce the first report.

Over the course of the time period that The Colorado Trust funded the CIP communities, the project directors became more and more committed to involving their community in selecting indicators and disseminating data. At the same time, they began to realize from direct personal experience that this could not be achieved with a linear process. In conversations with representatives of the CIP steering committee, the project directors criticized the original flow chart (Figure 3.3) as too limited and artificial. This criticism was formally acknowledged with a revamping of the process model. Namely, during one of the networking meetings, the project directors and the steering committee jointly produced the "meandering path" picture in Figure 3.5 as a more accurate depiction of the actual process that one needs to travel to develop an effective community indicators project.

Outcomes From Community Indicators Projects

REPORTS

Of the 15 communities funded by The Colorado Trust under CIP, 12 published and disseminated "indicators reports" as envisioned at the outset of the initiative. The formats of these reports varied from glossy, 16-page booklets; to more in-depth, 60-page, spiral-bound reports; to inserts in the local newspaper. In addition to producing these reports, some of the projects have posted indicator data on Web sites and created slide shows to present to organizations throughout the community.

Of the three projects that did not publish indicators reports, two developed lengthy draft versions but, due to staff turnover and funding constraints, were unable to finalize and publish their reports. The other project withdrew from the initiative before completing the CIP process (due to a decision by the local CHCI agency to disband the organization), but this project produced an interim report that was intended to set the stage for further work.

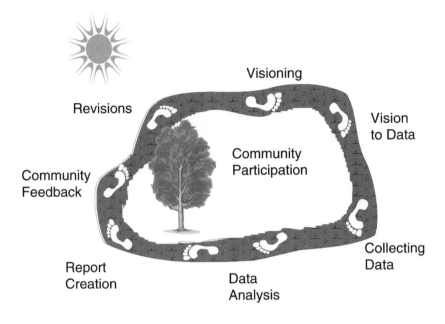

Figure 3.5   The "Meandering Path" Framework for Developing Community Indicators

COMMUNITY CHANGE

Although the physical report serves as the primary "product" of an indicators process, the ultimate "payoff" for the project is the potential it offers to change local decision making and to improve the health and well-being of the community. These outcomes are possible if the indicators report actually becomes a source of information for key decision makers in the public, nonprofit, and/or private sectors by pointing out to them which issues deserve their attention and by helping them to understand the systemwide impacts of their actions.

This change process inevitably requires time and patience, even under the best of circumstances (i.e., strong community buy-in, an informative high-profile report, sophisticated use of the data, and strategic targeting of key audiences). In at least some of the CIP communities, the indicators reports did garner public attention and stimulate changes in policy, practice, or conceptualization. The following are a few examples:

- The Mesa Civic Forum's "Our Picture of Health" publicized the need for public transportation and laid the groundwork for the county's first transit system.
- Indicator data have been used by nonprofit organizations and United Ways in some CIP communities in their strategic planning and budgeting decisions.

- The indicator projects in several CIP communities have brought diverse community-based organizations together around a common framework to collaborate on projects and to write joint grant proposals.
- Town councils and community foundations in some CIP communities revised their funding priorities in line with the issues highlighted by indicators reports.

A particularly noteworthy, albeit unique, example of an indicators-induced impact occurred in the OHC project, described earlier, with regard to the data reported on "livable wages." According to calculations in the indicators report, a single person with no children would need to earn at least $8.74 per hour to "sustain a healthy household" within that region of the state. After reviewing these data, two locally based banks raised their starting salaries from $7.50 to $9.00 per hour. According to the vice president for human relations at one of the banks, "That document was the key." A representative of the other bank remarked, "Employers around town are beginning to see what they have to pay their employees if they want them to stay." Indeed, there is evidence that other firms in the area also improved their pay scales and benefits packages (Porter-Norton, 1999).

In those communities where the indicators reports succeeded in stimulating elected officials and organizations to take action or to conduct business differently, the CHCI organization that housed the indicators projects tended to gain some collateral benefit. In effect, a successful community indicators project helped the respective CHCI groups to define in concrete terms what the "healthy communities" approach actually involves (e.g., a holistic approach to understanding health, broad-based community participation, bringing diverse segments together around a common vision, using systems thinking to find strategic leverage points). For CHCI projects such as OHC, Healthy Mountain Communities, and Yampa Valley Partners, community indicators became an essential component of their organizational identity and programmatic strategy (Larson, Christian, Olson, Hicks, & Sweeney, 2002).

EXTENSION OF THE COMMUNITY INDICATORS APPROACH ACROSS COLORADO

Community indicators were spotlighted by the Colorado Center for Healthy Communities, the organization responsible for creating a network among the various healthy communities projects that had been funded under CHCI.[8] In its newsletter, the center promoted indicators as

a significant opportunity for Healthy Communities if they are used well. In an era of information overload, indicators can stand out as crystallizing statements. . . . When used skillfully, indicators can encourage a community into action and produce powerful outcomes. (Fay, 1999, p. 3)

In addition to the 15 CHCI projects that were funded under CIP, two other projects have embarked on community indicators with funding from the Colorado Center for Healthy Communities as well as local matching funds. The Summit County CHCI project produced its first indicators report in 2000. The Peak-to-Peak Healthy Communities Project began the process of selecting indicators in 2000.

In addition to encouraging more CHCI projects to develop their own indicators, the Colorado Center for Healthy Communities promoted a state-level indicators project in August 2000. According to the center's announcement of this project, the objective was to "explore, identify, and research indicators that measure and track factors affecting the quality of life in Colorado and use them to develop a preliminary index of the state's quality of life." The center has been interested in creating an index that could influence policymaking at the statewide level in the same way that localized indicators reports guided community-level decision making.

As the Colorado Center for Healthy Communities and the individual CIP projects pursued their indicators work in more depth, they began to find overlap with the efforts of state agencies. The state demographer looked to the CIP projects as a mechanism for helping local officials and citizens to make better use of the data available through his office. He also played an active role in supporting the state-level index project.

Another example is the Interagency Prevention Council (IAPC), a task force of agency heads convened by the governor to create a coordinated strategy for funding risk reduction programs (e.g., substance abuse, violence, child abuse) throughout state government. The IAPC reached out to the CIP communities as a means of bringing grassroots input into its process. Representatives from 10 of the 15 CIP projects took part in a series of meetings that established a conceptual framework for the IAPC indicators and recommended 33 specific indicators. A change in governors led to institutional restructuring (i.e., the IAPC was folded into a new division within the Department of Public Health and the Environment), which in turn caused the indicators framework to be discarded in favor of a loose-knit list of 170 disparate indicators. At the time this chapter was being written, however, it appeared that the division's new director was interested in resurrecting the IAPC framework because of its coherence and grassroots input.

SUSTAINABILITY OF
COMMUNITY INDICATORS PROJECTS

In designing CIP, The Colorado Trust believed that it would be possible for projects to produce two annual reports within the 2-year funding time frame. Ideally, two annual reports would establish enough local interest and credibility to attract funding to sustain the process in perpetuity (akin to the Jacksonville model). In practice, however, most CIP grantees published their first reports during the waning months of their grants.

Of the 12 CIP grantees that produced reports under their grants, at least half actively worked to update their data at a later point in time. By July 2001, five grantees (Boulder, Healthy Mountain Communities, OHC, Pueblo, and Yampa Valley) had produced follow-up reports, and one other site (Mesa) was in the process of updating its report.[9] The sites that are still actively engaged in indicators work are relying much more on the World Wide Web as a medium for disseminating the data. This technology reduces the cost of producing and distributing reports while also making it easy to update the reports as new data become available.[10]

Lack of funding has been the primary obstacle for those CIP grantees whose indicators work ended with their first reports. Without support for the CIP project directors, many CHCI sites found it very difficult to sustain the process, particularly the more costly steps of updating data, presenting findings, and convening stakeholders to revisit the choice of indicators. It should also be noted that many of the local CHCI organizations faced tenuous funding situations with regard to their own survival, and this made it difficult to find the resources to support individual programs such as community indicators. (On the other hand, as pointed out earlier, investing in a community indicators program provides one means by which a healthy communities organization can identify its purpose and stake out its niche.)

In at least one case, a local indicators project was allowed to "die" (or at least to go dormant) because the community did not react to the report as the project staff had hoped. In this rural community, the indicators report was angrily denounced by a county commissioner during the initial unveiling. He argued that the report identified too many negative trends (e.g., crime, lack of services) and that this suggested that the commissioners might not be doing a good job. This experience provided the project staff with a painful lesson about local politics, as well as about the power of data, and this discouraged them from pursuing the dissemination effort any further.

ASSESSMENT OF INITIATIVE

CIP did not include a formal evaluation component. Instead, the CIP steering committee monitored the status of the initiative through periodic interactions with grantees during site visits, phone conversations, and networking meetings. In addition, the evaluator of the overarching CHCI, Ross Conner, extended his evaluation to include CIP as well, although the scope of the CIP assessment was inherently much less comprehensive than that of the CHCI evaluation due to budget constraints. In addition to participating in the ongoing monitoring process of the CIP steering committee, he conducted formal interviews with the first eight CIP project directors and held informal discussions with the other seven project directors. This section describes a set of findings that emerged during the CIP assessment process.

In a general sense, it is clear from the interviews and conversations that the participating communities generally found a great deal of value in the community indicators approach. At the same time, the project directors and their communities learned many valuable lessons about what it takes to conduct an effective indicators project. These can be grouped into four categories: the larger context surrounding a CIP project, the general process of conducting the project, the community's response to indicators reports, and longer term outcomes from the project.

Larger Context

Because CIP so explicitly emphasized the need for broad community participation, the projects necessarily needed to acknowledge and respond to the larger community context. For many projects, the local advisory committee provided a vital linkage to the different sectors and interests that influence local affairs. In addition to bringing information and values into the project, the advisory committee provided a buffer against political or agency pressures. For instance, in decisions about the selection or deletion of particular indicators, CIP committees helped to shield the project from parochial interests, allowing the indicator set to be more fully anchored in the consensus vision of a healthy community. The advisory group could also provide a liaison benefit by explaining the purpose and benefits of the indicators project to the general public.

Another important aspect of the community context was the larger CHCI planning and implementation process within which the CIP effort existed. Many CIP projects were also connected to additional community-based strategic planning efforts in the areas of land use, economic development, and social service reform. It was important for the CIP projects to find common ground with these other initiatives and to include representatives in the development of indicators. In some cases, the CIP project director actually provided direct support to the other initiatives to help them achieve their own objectives. As the CIP process became more inclusive and sensitive to these other initiatives, it took more time to work through the various steps of developing indicators.

The Process of Developing Indicators

The involvement of many stakeholders in the indicator selection process significantly prolonged the period of time required to produce the first report. In many cases, the working group repeatedly revisited its list of indicators as new members joined the group and new ideas were floated. This process of indicator selection might appear inefficient to most researchers, but the extended period of community involvement was crucial for increasing the community's acceptance of the project and its willingness to use the data. The point of CIP was to generate data and reports that would influence how local residents and organizations see and act toward their community. At the very least, this requires widespread input into the question of what to measure and ongoing community-wide conversations about what the data mean.

In terms of specific lessons related to the indicator development process, the project directors most frequently reported the following:

- The process should be question driven, not data driven. The vision provides a framework that leads to a question-focused process (e.g., "Is our community meeting the transportation needs of our residents?") rather than reverting to a data-driven process (e.g., "Data about car usage are available from the state, so we will include them in our set").
- In working with subcommittees or citizens groups to solicit input on dimensions and possible indicators, go to where they are and meet them on "their turf" to get the best input and acceptance.
- Having examples of actual completed indicators reports from many different communities helps to make the process concrete for participants and also provides new ideas.
- Establishing a clear set of steps and a tentative schedule for the process helps to start and keep the work on track. Be prepared to make adjustments, however, particularly to the schedule. As one director said, "Everything seems to take longer than expected." There was an important related lesson: Deadlines are "painful but useful."
- Having some "demand-driven" members on the advisory committee is useful in anchoring the process. By this, project directors mean people who were focused less on technical data issues than on the ultimate purpose and utility of the measures. The mix of data-driven and demand-driven perspectives resulted in the best compromises in the final selection of indicators.

Community Response to Indicators Reports

Nearly all of the organizations funded under CIP published reports and disseminated indicator data to the larger community. Taken together, these experiences demonstrate that community indicators can capture the attention—and sometimes even the imagination—of local residents and officials. If these reports are to make a real difference in the way in which people think and act, however, the data must have real meaning. The following lessons relate to the process of translating data into meaningful information:

- Indicators, in and of themselves, do not tell a story. They need a framework, such as a vision, that unites them and can be used to explain their meaning.

- Although a written report is important, the "story" of the indicators can be best told in presentations around the community. This increases public interest in the indicators and in their use.
- In many (but not all) cases, the CIP process and products created a desire for more and better data about different aspects of the community.

Longer Term Outcomes

The major evaluation issue with regard to CIP is whether the indicators reports actually made a difference as to the decisions and behavior of local residents and officials. The "livable wage" story from OHC provides a vivid example of the type of impact that is possible; however, most of the other "success stories" are more subtle. Rather than reporting a single indicator that compels readers to act differently, the more typical impact is the case where the indicators report leads elected officials and community leaders to begin focusing on hidden or underappreciated issues. As attention is drawn to new issues or to connections between issues, the public agenda begins to shift and resources are devoted to new "solutions." In other words, the most likely mechanism for indicators projects to improve a community's health and well-being is to foster among (at least some) residents a higher level of awareness regarding local health status and then to maintain a focus on critical issues until conditions improve.

This consciousness-raising approach is very much in keeping with the philosophy underlying healthy communities. Rather than advocating a particular ideologically based policy, the CHCI projects have typically worked toward deeper and more inclusive analysis of key community issues. In at least a few of the communities (Mesa County, OHC, and Yampa Valley), the project directors deliberately established a conceptual framework for their indicators reports that would promote "systems thinking," efficient solutions, and/or sustainable development (AtKisson, 1996; Farrell & Hart, 1998; Meadows, 1998). This approach requires receptivity, analysis, and a certain degree of sophistication on the part of the target audience. Some communities are more open to this level of intervention than are others. Even in those communities where the key decision makers are receptive, it takes time and ongoing reinforcement for community conversations to become open, inclusive of multiple perspectives, and holistic.

Conclusion

The CIP experience demonstrated that most communities are able to undertake the complex process of determining how to measure health and quality of life (with or without the technical research capacity of a local university) and to produce reports that convey meaningful data to different audiences in the community. Before people are willing to move to action, however, they must answer questions such as the following:

- Which indicators are the most vital to focus on?
- Why are these indicators going up (or down)?
- Where should this community be on each of these indicators?
- What sorts of actions would move these indicators in the right direction?

None of these questions has an absolute answer; they all hinge on a community's underlying values, current realities, and opportunities. A community indicators project can generate answers and thus motivate behavior by provoking deep community-wide conversations. Data can provide a relatively objective starting point for these community conversations; people living and working in the community then can delve deeper into the realities that underlie the statistical picture and the steps that are necessary to change it.

Notes

1. The Colorado Trust did provide funding for a group of "expert" advisers who had experience in starting up other indicators projects, but these individuals all reinforced the philosophy that each community needs to decide for itself how to measure "community health."

2. The initiative was designed to help communities promote health in two distinct ways: (a) by introducing a comprehensive inclusive approach to strategic planning that would identify critical action steps and (b) by providing a forum in which residents could develop skills, leadership, relationships, and a consensus decision-making process that would continue to pay off as the community faced new health-related issues in the future.

3. Another factor underlying The Colorado Trust's interest in supporting community indicators was the potential value that such indicators might serve for the evaluation of CHCI. Because the CHCI projects all adopted their own key performance areas and action plans, there could be no uniform criteria for evaluating the "success" of the different grantees. Community indicators offered the possibility of tracking each grantee's progress according to those dimensions of "health" that the community regarded as most important and relevant to local conditions (Conner, Tanjasiri, Davidson, Dempsey, & Robles, 1998).

4. These outside speakers included Alan AtKisson (Sustainable Seattle and Redefining Progress), Craig Freshly (Maine Economic Growth Council), Deborah Silver (Pasadena [California] Public Health Department), and David Swain (Jacksonville [Florida] Community Council Inc.).

5. This case study is based largely on interviews with the OHC project director, Lynn Shine.

6. In addition to the three counties that make up the official OHC region (Archuleta, La Plata, and San Juan), the OHC project gathered data for neighboring Dolores County. Dolores County was added to meet the needs of the stakeholders from the U.S. Forest Service who were developing a plan for San Juan National Forest (which extends into Dolores County).

7. None of the CIP grantees actually succeeded in measuring spirituality, although two (Boulder County and Montezuma County) referenced this domain in their reports. Because of the grantees' interest in measuring spirituality, The Colorado Trust subcontracted with a consultant to develop a group process that would lead to an operational definition of "spirituality" (Grace, 1999).

8. The Colorado Healthy Communities Council changed its name to the Colorado Center for Healthy Communities in 1999. With financial support primarily from The Colorado Trust, the organization had a paid staff from 1996 through April 2001, at which point the organization reverted to an all-volunteer networking group staffed by local CHCI directors.

9. Information about more recent CIP activities was provided by Colin Laird, director of Healthy Mountain Communities in Carbondale.

10. For examples of Web-based indicators reports produced by CIP grantees, see www.bococivicforum.org, www.hmccolorado.org, and www.yampavalleypartners.com.

References

Andrews, J. H. (1996, September). Going by the numbers. *Planning*, pp. 14–18.

Ashton, J. (Ed.). (1992). *Healthy cities*. Milton Keynes, UK: Open University Press.

AtKisson, A. (1996). Developing indicators of sustainable community: Lessons from Sustainable Seattle. *Environmental Impact Assessment Review, 16*, 337–350.

Besleme, K., Maser, E., & Silverstein, J. (1999). *A community indicators case study: Addressing the quality of life in two communities*. San Francisco: Redefining Progress.

Besleme, K., & Mullin, M. (1997). Community indicators and healthy communities. *National Civic Review, 86*, 43–52.

Cobb, C.W., & Rixford, C. (1998). *Lessons learned from the history of social indicators*. San Francisco: Redefining Progress.

Conner, R. F., Tanjasiri, S. P., Davidson, M., Dempsey, C., & Robles, G. (1998). *Citizens making their communities healthier: A description of the Colorado Healthy Communities Initiative*. Denver: The Colorado Trust.

Farrell, A., & Hart, M. (1998). What does sustainability really mean? The search for useful indicators. *Environment, 40*(9), 4–9, 26–31.

Fay, K. (1999, Winter). What are indicators? *Pathways: A Publication of the Colorado Center for Healthy Communities*, p. 3.

Gahin, R., & Paterson, C. (2001). Community indicators: Past, present, and future. *National Civic Review, 90*, 347–361.

Grace, J. (1999). *Indicators of healthy communities in the domain of spirituality*. Denver: The Colorado Trust.

Gross, B. M., & Straussman, J. D. (1974). The social indicators movement. *Social Policy, 5*, 43–54.

Hancock, T., & Duhl, L. (1986). *Healthy cities: Promoting health in the urban context* (World Health Organization Healthy Cities Papers No. 1). Copenhagen, Denmark: FADL Publishers.

Innes, J. (1990). *Knowledge and public policy: The search for meaningful indicators*. New Brunswick, NJ: Transaction Publishers.

Jacksonville Community Council Inc. (2001). *Quality of life in Jacksonville: Indicators for progress*. Jacksonville, FL: Author.

Kickbusch, I. (1989). Healthy cities: A working movement and a growing project. *Health Promotion International, 4*, 77–82.

Kretzmann, J., & McKnight, J. (1993). *Building communities from the inside out: A path toward finding and mobilizing a community's assets*. Chicago: ACTA Publications.

Land, K. (1992). Social indicators. In E. F. Borgatta & M. L. Borgatta (Eds.), *The encyclopedia of sociology*. New York: Macmillan.

Larson, C., Christian, A., Olson, L., Hicks, D., & Sweeney, C. (2002). *Colorado Healthy Communities Initiative: Ten years later*. Denver: The Colorado Trust.

Meadows, D. (1993, May 22). Using salmon runs and gardens to measure our well-being. *Valley News* (Lebanon, NH), p. 24.

Meadows, D. (1998). *Indicators and information systems for sustainable development* (report to the Balaton Group). Hartland Four Corners, VT: Sustainability Institute.

Operation Healthy Communities. (1997). *Pathways to healthier communities: Archuleta, Dolores, La Plata, and San Juan Counties.* Durango, CO: Author.

Porter-Norton, M. (1999, Winter). Indicators to action: Livable wages in southwest Colorado. *Pathways: A Publication of the Colorado Center for Healthy Communities,* pp. 4–5.

Redefining Progress, Tyler Norris Associates, & Sustainable Seattle. (1997). *The community indicators handbook: Measuring progress toward healthy and sustainable communities.* San Francisco: Redefining Progress.

Smith, J. A. (1991). *The idea brokers: Think tanks and the rise of the new policy elite.* New York: Free Press.

Sustainable Seattle. (1995). *Indicators of sustainable community.* Seattle, WA: Author.

Wilkinson, R., & Marmot, M. (Eds.). (1998). *Social determinants of health: The solid facts.* Copenhagen, Denmark: World Health Organization, Regional Office for Europe.

World Health Organization. (1946). *Constitution.* New York: Author.

World Health Organization. (1986). *The Ottawa charter for health promotion.* Ottawa: Health and Welfare Canada.

4

The Teen Pregnancy Prevention 2000 Initiative

Community Building Through Consensus

Kaia M. Gallagher

Jodi G. Drisko

When health promotion projects are community based, communities become active participants in identifying problems, mobilizing resources, and developing strategies for how these problems should be solved (Minkler, 1997). Yet how easily are such initiatives undertaken for a topic such as teen pregnancy that by its nature generates controversy and dissent? Issues such as teen sexual activity, pregnancy, and childbearing inevitably result in debates regarding how these problems should be framed and, more particularly, how they should be solved, in most instances with no clear resolution being reached (National Campaign to Prevent Teen Pregnancy, 1998). Given the inability of communities to agree on the parameters of why teen pregnancy is occurring, local teen pregnancy prevention interventions can appear diffuse and appear unfocused. Nonetheless, participants in these projects have been found to judge their efforts to be successful in (a) *reaching consensus* on areas where agreement can be achieved, (b) *increasing community awareness* of a problem that is frequently ignored or denied, and (c) *developing community resources* to meet the needs of youth and families. As measures of a community's ability to respond to problems such as teen pregnancy, these would appear to be critical first steps, but how connected are these activities to teen pregnancy prevention?

The purpose of this chapter is to review the results of the Teen Pregnancy Prevention 2000 Initiative (TPPI), a 5-year demonstration project that lasted between 1993 and 1998 in the state of Colorado. TPPI was well funded, expending $7.7 million over 5 years within five grantee communities. In establishing this initiative, The Colorado Trust permitted its grantee communities to choose for themselves the types of programs they wanted to adopt to address teen pregnancy; in addition, the foundation provided each grantee community $50,000 per year over 4 years to implement its proposed projects. Similar to other community-based initiatives that have focused on teen pregnancy,[1] TPPI was designed by The Colorado Trust to contain several key project components. During the first year of the project, the grantee communities were required to develop strategic implementation plans without being given an explicit prevention model to follow. Diverse stakeholders had to be included as part of the planning process, and these stakeholders were expected to reach consensus regarding the implementation strategies that would be funded by the initiative.

This chapter summarizes the outcomes resulting from TPPI as an example of community-based teen pregnancy prevention. A key issue is how "success" is defined from the perspective of the participating communities. Like other community-based initiatives, TPPI presents evaluation challenges in the broad range of outcomes that occurred, the evolving nature of the intervention, and the idiosyncratic manner in which the initiative was implemented in the five grantee communities (Connell, Kubisch, Schorr, & Weiss, 1995). At the same time, the results underscore the potential that community-based interventions offer in terms of increasing the capacity of communities to work together to solve their problems (Kreuter, Young, & Lezin, 1998; White & Whelage, 1995). The results also suggest a broader vantage point for understanding the mechanisms of teen pregnancy prevention from the perspective of community-level change.

Context: Teen Pregnancy as a Health Promotion Issue

Teen pregnancy, by definition a medical event, is also a social phenomenon deeply rooted in cultural, social, and community contexts. The wide variation in teen pregnancy rates among nations, regions, and racial/ethnic groups speaks to how social contexts define the circumstances under which teenagers become young mothers (Trussell, Card, & Hogue, 1998). Within the United States, group variations in teen pregnancy have been attributed to cultural definitions regarding how teen motherhood is valued. In African American neighborhoods where poverty is prevalent, teen motherhood can be seen as a "rite of passage" for teens who have few other perceivable options (Anderson, 1991; Dash, 1989). Early motherhood among Hispanics has been associated with norms associating motherhood as a desirable state as well as historic patterns of discrimination, limited educational attainment, and differing levels of acculturation (Brindis, 1992). The degree to which teens anticipate teen pregnancy to be a hardship has also been found to vary by socioeconomic class (Luker, 1996).

In addition to defining the "appropriateness" of teen pregnancy, certain community contexts have been found to "protect" adolescents against the risky behaviors that can lead to teen pregnancy. Communities that offer youth a "web of influence," uniting parents, teachers, religious leaders, and neighbors to help adolescents, can overcome the circumstances found in economically disadvantaged neighborhoods (Connell, Spencer, & Aber, 1994; Price, Cioci, Penner, & Trautlein, 1993). Substantial research also links family support, positive family communication, and parent involvement in schooling with higher youth self-esteem, lower amounts of risk taking, and improved school performance. Beyond family environments, the presence of caring schools, adults involved in the lives of youth, and supportive neighborhoods has been shown to promote fewer behavior problems among youth, a lower incidence of risk-taking behaviors, improved self-image, and greater hopes for the future (Scales & Leffert, 1999).

Complementing these contextual approaches, traditional teen pregnancy programs have been developed that deal directly with personal behaviors and choices. Programs of this type include Postponing Sexual Involvement (Howard & McCabe, 1992), the Reducing the Risk sexuality education curriculum (Card, Brindis, Paterson, & Niego, 1999), and school-based reproductive health services (Zabin, 1992).

Despite the multiplicity of programs designed to address the teen pregnancy problem, experience has shown that teen pregnancy has "no easy answers" and that no single solution can be readily applied to all community settings (Frost & Forrest, 1995; Institute of Medicine, 1995; Kirby, 1997; Miller, Card, Paikoff, & Peterson, 1992; Philiber & Namerow, 1995). Programs designed to produce individual-level change have been found to do so by (a) reducing sexual behaviors that lead to unintended pregnancies; (b) incorporating behavioral goals that are age, experience, and culturally appropriate; (c) relying on proven theories of change; (d) lasting long enough to have an effect; (e) providing accurate information; (f) using a variety of teaching methods; (g) addressing social pressures to have sex; (h) providing models in communication; and (i) using trainers who believe in the program (Kirby, 1997).

Community-Based
Approaches to Teen Pregnancy Prevention

Given the fact that teen pregnancy is not a straightforward issue that lends itself to clearly defined solutions, funders and government agencies have begun to employ community-based approaches for defining and resolving the problem in a locally relevant way. Evaluations of community-based health promotion efforts show that this type of health promotion strategy can be time-consuming and process intensive (Bruner, 1991) and is not always successful. Altman et al. (1991) point out that up to half of all coalitions dissolve within their first year of operation because they cannot accomplish the basic tasks of forming coalitions. Community members who participate in these endeavors often come to the process unfamiliar with the work to be done, the processes to be followed, and the ways in which they might work as equals with the professional participants (Kotloff, Roaf, & Gambone, 1995). Moreover, some evaluations have found that having community members involved in health promotion initiatives can slow program development, conflict with efficient program operations, and serve to create program goals that differ from the programs' original goals (Howell, Devaney, McCormick, & Raykovich, 1998).

Case reports from the New Futures initiative, funded by the Annie E. Casey Foundation, point out the difficulties that community coalitions have in dealing with teen pregnancy prevention. Members of the coalitions funded under the New Futures program decided to provide access to information and contraception so as to reduce teen pregnancy rates, only to find that teen pregnancy rates actually increased after these policies were adopted. Another stumbling block faced by some of the coalitions was unresolved discussions regarding the merits of particular sex education curricula. Failure to reach consensus about the appropriateness of various programs stymied the ability of these coalitions to identify prevention strategies acceptable to all group members (White & Whelage, 1995).

Similar experiences have been reported within communities funded under the Plain Talk initiative by the Annie E. Casey Foundation. During an initial planning year, groups of community stakeholders were expected to reach consensus regarding implementation strategies for teen pregnancy prevention. Communities that experienced the most difficulty were those with larger numbers of stakeholders who were ethnic minorities or members of conservative religious groups, with some communities discovering that there were limits to the extent to which stakeholders with sharply opposing views could reconcile their differences (Kotloff et al., 1995).

Other studies of teen pregnancy prevention coalitions confirm that one of the most controversial issues faced by these groups is whether contraception should be available to adolescents and where and how it should be provided

(Institute of Medicine, 1995; Lawson & Rhode, 1993). A related issue is the extent to which parents should be informed about and/or consent to having their adolescents gain access to contraception. Recognizing the impossibility of reaching agreement on these issues, many coalitions focus on the importance of teen pregnancy as a problem, adopting strategies that involve information dissemination, the creation of resource inventories, and awareness-building strategies (Nezlek & Galano, 1993). Focusing on awareness building is an activity that can energize coalitions through increased visibility and by providing "quick wins," but many coalitions appear to be unable to move beyond awareness activities toward more focused programs that can result in observable changes in health status (Kreuter & Lezin, 1998).

In sum, although there is increasing recognition of the importance of mobilizing communities to address teen pregnancy prevention concerns, less is known about the characteristics of effective programs designed to promote community-level change. What is known is that teen pregnancy approaches need to be long term (Hutchins, 1999), inclusive of the values of communities in which they are being implemented (Card et al., 1999), and multidimensional, incorporating a wide variety of strategies (Philiber & Namerow, 1995). Unfortunately, the choices as to which strategies should be adopted are often complicated by the unwillingness of many community members to acknowledge that teen pregnancy is a problem, conflict surrounding the most appropriate strategies to adopt (National Campaign to Reduce Teen Pregnancy, 1997; Philiber & Namerow, 1995), and a lack of funding for large-scale community efforts (Howard & Mitchell, 1993; Schorr, 1988).

The Teen Pregnancy Prevention 2000 Initiative

The Teen Pregnancy Prevention 2000 Initiative adopted a community-based approach for defining and resolving teen pregnancy structured around collaboration, community consensus, and financial support for infrastructure and program development. In essence, this initiative had three characteristics that define it as community based: (a) the locus of decision making and control, (b) the overall intervention goals as uniquely developed in each grantee community, and (c) the support provided for resource/capacity development.

WHERE WAS THE LOCUS OF
DECISION MAKING AND CONTROL?

Within community-based projects, decision making can be viewed along a continuum from projects that are fully community determined to those in which the community is a more passive participant (Hancock et al., 1997). Within TPPI, The Colorado Trust chose to fund "community collaboratives that were in turn sponsored by a lead agency. The community collaboratives each employed a full-time project director and functioned within a different organizational setting; two community grantees created nonprofit agencies, whereas the three other grantees relied on parent agencies, operating in a semi-independent manner within a larger organizational context.

Within the grantee communities, the stakeholder groups that were formed during the first planning year were designed to be inclusive, bringing together all of the representative voices in the community. Efforts were made to ensure that all agency and service sector views were included. Stakeholders were also recruited from important subgroups within the community, with a particular emphasis on incorporating the views of youth themselves. In all, 332 participants were involved in some part of the stakeholder process across the six communities originally funded. The total number of stakeholders involved ranged from 135 to 142 participants on a yearly basis. Of these, nearly a third (29%) were community members without any direct agency or organizational connection to teen pregnancy.

WHAT WERE THE OVERALL GOALS OF THE INTERVENTIONS DEVELOPED BY THE GRANTEE COMMUNITIES?

As part of the first-year planning activities, the TPPI grantee communities were asked to develop their visions as to the types of change that would occur in their communities. Professional facilitators worked with the communities over a series of successive meetings to help communities define how they envisioned a successful teen pregnancy prevention campaign. TPPI grantees were also provided with technical assistance on teen risk behaviors and effective teen pregnancy prevention programs as they were developing their first-year plans. The visions developed by the grantees show the types of community-level change toward which the communities were collectively directed. In particular, a content analysis of the vision statements revealed three themes common to the five grantee communities:

1. Community settings need to be supportive of the needs of families and youth.

2. Strengthening families is an important concomitant of helping youth.

3. Communities can offer a positive vision for youth that in turn will encourage healthy decision making, empowerment, and hope for the future.

From the beginning, the TPPI grantee communities were aiming their collective efforts toward community-level change as a more indirect strategy for changing the individual behaviors that are the antecedents of teen pregnancy. While sharing common visions with the other grantee communities, each community also developed an individualized plan with different target goals and objectives, most of which retained a focus on community-level awareness building and resource development. Because these projects were also funded to provide case management to pregnant and parenting teens, some communities chose to establish supplemental programs for high-risk and parenting teens (e.g., support groups, mentoring programs).

WHAT WAS THE LEVEL OF SUPPORT PROVIDED TO THE GRANTEE COMMUNITIES FOR RESOURCE AND CAPACITY DEVELOPMENT?

As a community-directed intervention, TPPI benefited from generous funding over its 5-year duration. Each project received sufficient support to sustain a full-time project director, administrative support staff, two case managers, and (during the final years) a part-time resource developer. In addition, supplemental funds were made available for each project to hire a part-time local evaluator as well as to receive technical assistance in the areas of facilitation, strategic planning, needs assessment, case management development, and fund development.

Believing in the communities' ability to define for themselves the most appropriate strategies for teen pregnancy prevention, The Colorado Trust empowered the grantees to develop their individual strategic plans without defining a priori what components should be included. Further in accord with this "no interference" policy, the projects were given $50,000 per year for 4 years without limits imposed by the funder.

Community-Based Initiatives Characterized by This Initiative

Table 4.1 summarizes the key activities defined by the TPPI project directors as their communities' accomplishments (Gallagher & Drisko, 1998). The range of activities listed underscores the changes toward which the five TPPI communities directed their efforts and resources, including programs for youth, families, and the community broadly defined. This listing provides a composite view of the strategic directions that evolved within the TPPI grantee communities based on the consensus reached by the respective stakeholder groups.

Table 4.1   Major Accomplishments Within Each TPPI Community

Community	Accomplishments

Arvada	Community Education Efforts
	  – Parents Count (parent curriculum teaching children about sexuality)
	  – RETHINK anger management classes
	  – Youth asset development forums
	  – "Baby Think It Over" dolls
	Activities for Teens
	  – Teen center established
	  – Coupon books for "in-need" youth
	  – Community service programs
	Services for Youth
	  – Mentoring programs
	  – Counseling case management services

Aurora	Support Programs for Pregnant, Parenting, and At-Risk Youth
	  – Activity groups for at-risk teens
	  – Male responsibility groups
	  – Parenting classes
	  – Support groups
	  – Low-income housing program
	Prevention Curriculum Implemented in the Aurora Public Schools
	  – Male/Female team teaching program titled "It Takes Two"

Colorado Springs	Services for Pregnant and At-Risk Youth
	  – InterCept program for high-risk middle school youth
	  – Go Girl program for high-risk high school youth
	  – Abstinence education
	  – Non-Couples program for teen parents
	Activities for Teens
	  – Teen newspaper
	  – Teen center
	  – "Toast to Teens" recognition program
	Services for Families
	  – Master Teacher program to train community educators
	  – First Visitor program offering home visitation to new parents
	  – Parenting training

Delta-Montrose	Services for Pregnant, Parenting, and At-Risk Youth
	  – Charter school for pregnant and parenting girls
	  – Mentoring/Counseling program for at-risk middle school youth
	  – Youth yellow pages

Table 4.1   (Continued)

Community	Accomplishments

	Activities for Youth
	  – Mini-Grant program for recreation and other
	    community projects
	  – Youth assets survey and campaign
	  – Peer counseling program
	Community Activities
	  – Community of Caring program in seven schools

West Denver	Community Projects
	  – Funding for 10 locally defined programs and
	    services per year
	  – Brochures on community strategies for preventing
	    teen pregnancy
	  – Fliers on the link between sexual abuse and
	    teen pregnancy

As comprehensive as this list of TPPI accomplishments is, there are also other types of teen pregnancy prevention interventions that these community-based projects did *not* include. In 1987, the Institute of Medicine identified three types of teen pregnancy prevention efforts that have been proven to be effective: (a) those that impart knowledge or influence attitudes, (b) those that provide access to contraception, and (c) those that enhance life options (Hayes, 1987). Although all five of the grantee communities developed programs that could be classified as either "imparting knowledge/changing attitudes" or "enhancing life options," none addressed "access to contraception." Key informant interviews with the TPPI project directors suggest that contraception was not a topic on which the stakeholder groups within the grantee communities could reach consensus. This failure to reach consensus can be attributed in part to beliefs among some of the stakeholders that providing access to contraception is not an effective means to prevent teen pregnancy, as revealed in a stakeholder survey conducted during the second year of the project.

A total of 234 surveys were mailed to all stakeholders identified as having been associated with one of the five TPPI grantee projects. Of these surveys, 57.6% were returned, with a response rate that varied by community between 54% and 69%. Respondents were broadly reflective of the stakeholder membership; a quarter of the surveys (25.2%) were returned by community members, with the remainder being completed by educators, health care providers, and other service providers. Analysis of the nonresponders revealed that many had not attended recent TPPI meetings and appeared to have dropped out of their respective stakeholder groups.

Within the survey, the stakeholders were asked about their views on the factors associated with teen pregnancy. Slightly more than half (54%) identified "contraceptive unavailability" as influencing teen pregnancy. In comparison, there was much stronger agreement among the stakeholders regarding 12 other factors as contributors to teen pregnancy: dropping out of school (96%), alcohol (96%), self-esteem (95%), sexual abuse (92%), hopeless future (91%), economics/poverty (88%), family history (88%), teens' denial (77%), adults' denial (71%), lack of knowledge regarding pregnancy risks (61%), welfare (59%), and lack of morals (55%). When asked to compare a variety of teen pregnancy prevention strategies, more than a quarter of the respondents (27%) actually regarded contraceptive availability as having "no impact" or as being "counterproductive."

These attitudes help to explain why the strategic plans developed by the five TPPI communities omitted "contraceptive availability" as a designated approach. With a quarter of the stakeholders not fully supporting this type of intervention as being effective in reducing teen pregnancy, consensus became difficult to achieve, eliminating contraception as a program that would be included in the strategic plans. Similar difficulties were experienced in some of the groups when sexuality education options were considered. Programs dealing with communication skills both for teens and for parents were, nonetheless, accepted by stakeholders in some communities.

Outcomes

WAS TPPI A SUCCESS AS A
COMMUNITY-BASED HEALTH PROMOTION PROJECT?

To evaluate the success of TPPI, a survey was sent to all participants to determine what they believed the outcomes to be of this 5-year collaborative effort. A total of 230 surveys were mailed to stakeholders who had been involved with TPPI over the previous 3 years, and a second mailing was sent to stakeholders who had not responded within 2 weeks supplemented by follow-up phone calls. A total of 76% of the surveys were returned, with a response rate that ranged between 70% and 81% among the five communities. Respondents indicated that they had been involved with the TPPI projects for an average of 3 years, with 60% having participated in the first-year planning activities.

Stakeholders were asked to report their perceptions relative to different types of community impacts. As shown in Table 4.2, the stakeholders can be seen as strongly agreeing that TPPI had positive community impacts in three areas: (a) increases in community awareness of and involvement in teen pregnancy prevention, (b) the development of programs and resources that would

Table 4.2   Stakeholder Views Regarding the Positive Outcomes of TPPI
($N = 175$)

Community Benefits of TPPI	Percentage "Strongly Agreeing" or "Somewhat Agreeing"
Increased community awareness of teen pregnancy	84.4
Increased number of people involved in this issue	82.6
Increased community dialogue about teen pregnancy	80.2
Increased media attention to this issue	68.1
Increased willingness of people to work together around this issue	77.7

serve youth and families, and (c) more generally, collaboration both within and outside of the coalitions.

TO WHAT EXTENT DID COMMUNITY AWARENESS OF TEEN PREGNANCY INCREASE IN THE TPPI COMMUNITIES?

Early within TPPI, stakeholders acknowledged in a survey that they believed that apathy and denial toward teen pregnancy were pervasive problems in each of the grantee communities (Research and Evaluation, Drisko, & Gallagher, 1995). Activities included in the strategic plans directly responded to the need to promote greater awareness of teen pregnancy within the project communities, and indeed a review of the progress reports from the five grantee sites confirms that a substantial amount of effort was placed on increasing the public's awareness of teen pregnancy using a wide array of media outlets. In addition, the project directors from all five sites developed a statewide media campaign encouraging parents to talk to their teens about sex. As part of this campaign, more than 10,000 guidebooks for facilitating parent-teen discussions were distributed. Stakeholders strongly agreed that by the final year of the project, community awareness of teen pregnancy did increase as a result of these efforts.

TO WHAT EXTENT DID RESOURCES FOR YOUTH AND FAMILIES INCREASE IN THE TPPI COMMUNITIES?

Building resources for youth was an early priority in each of the TPPI communities, with a lack of "recreation" services being identified as a particular

Table 4.3   Number of Programs Established or Funded Through TPPI: 1996

Program Focus	Arvada	Aurora	Colorado Springs	Delta-Montrose	West Denver
Related to teen pregnancy	4	7	3	5	1
Serving youth	22	13	5	34	11
Serving families	2		3	5	6
Serving the community		3		4	2

problem. In contrast, more traditional teen pregnancy strategies, such as providing greater access to family planning and improving comprehensive health education, were less commonly viewed as service gaps. Focus groups held with parents in each of the five grantee communities during the projects' third year further confirmed the need for additional youth- and family-centered recreation programs. One of the primary recommendations made by these groups was that additional resources be made available to support affordable activities for youth and families, including recreation, sports, family-oriented programs, and parenting classes (Research and Evaluation, Drisko, & Gallagher, 1997).

The programs developed through TPPI can be seen as a response to the need for additional youth- and family-oriented programs as defined by the community. As shown in Table 4.3, a wide variety of programs established or funded through TPPI served not only teens at risk for pregnancy but all youth, families, and the community as a whole. In fact, in all grantee communities, programs serving all youth outnumbered those targeted more specifically toward teens at risk for pregnancy.

The full impacts of these programs are difficult to capture. The stakeholders themselves, however, affirmed that the development of community-oriented programs was one of the lasting contributions of TPPI, as shown in Table 4.4. The provision of services for teen mothers and their infants through the case management was also acknowledged as a positive outcome of the initiative.

TO WHAT EXTENT DID COLLABORATION INCREASE IN THE TPPI COMMUNITIES?

One of the unique features of TPPI was its emphasis on using community "collaboratives" as the vehicle for promoting community change. Analysis of attendance patterns at TPPI meetings show that stakeholders from diverse backgrounds participated in TPPI meetings. In both the second year and the

Table 4.4   Stakeholder Views Regarding the Programmatic Outcomes of TPPI
               ($N = 175$)

Benefits of TPPI	Percentage "Strongly Agreeing" or "Somewhat Agreeing"
Expanded type and amount of services for teen moms	91.4
Expanded type and amount of services for infants of teens	76.6
Increased quality of health services for pregnant teens	80.8
Provided more activities for youth in the community	73.8
Increased the number of programs/services for youth	86.2

Table 4.5   Stakeholder Views Regarding Other Positive Outcomes of TPPI
               ($N = 175$)

Benefits of TPPI	Percentage "Strongly Agreeing" or "Somewhat Agreeing"
Increased awareness of other resources	71.0
Increased awareness of other collaborators	78.8

fifth year, stakeholders consistently reported in separate surveys that the development of professional and personal contacts through TPPI was a benefit of their participation (Table 4.5).

Open-ended comments by the stakeholders further confirm the value they place on their collaborative experience. Following are a few examples:

- "I believe the biggest impact has been the community collaboration and input."
- "It has brought the community together through cooperation."
- "I feel the concept of coalitions is extremely important in the future as the needs and monetary demands for community agencies increase. Coalitions provide vast benefits for the pooling of varied resources, multidisciplinary approaches to issues, avoidance of duplication of services, increased awareness of services, etc."

Above and beyond the personal benefits of collaboration, TPPI was able to mobilize other agencies to develop cooperative ventures related to youth issues. Given the difficulties associated with sustaining community coalitions, the fact that all five communities maintained their community-based stakeholder groups throughout the project's 5-year life is an accomplishment in itself. Kreuter has suggested that, above and beyond survival, community-based coalitions go through stages that include (a) preformation, (b) formation, (c) implementation/maintenance, and (d) reaching the point at which they are capable of achieving outcomes (Kreuter & Lezin, 1998). The TPPI collaboratives all were able to reach the fourth stage of coalition development due to project leadership and sustained funding support.

DID THE PROJECT STRENGTHEN THE DEVELOPMENT OF COMMUNITY CAPACITY?

TPPI was a community-directed intervention that received generous funding support over a relatively lengthy period of time. The projects were well staffed with full-time project directors, administrative support staff, two case managers, and (during the final years) a part-time resource developer. Support for a local evaluator was also made available, as was technical assistance in the areas of facilitation, strategic planning, needs assessment, case management development, and fund development. These resources provided an immediate base of personnel and financial support to the projects.

Although the projects were managed on a day-to-day basis by a full-time project director, stakeholder groups continued to provide direction and oversight throughout the lives of the projects. Whereas during the first year, large representative groups were recruited to provide input into the planning process, during later years, stakeholders functioned like boards of directors, typically meeting either monthly or quarterly to review the progress and direction of the activities being implemented. Members of these smaller steering committees typically were volunteers who chose to continue with the projects. In addition, the larger stakeholder bodies were reconvened on an annual basis in most communities. In terms of implementation, the projects conformed in their overall structure to the original 5-year plans developed by the community-based stakeholders.

Both individual and collective benefits were realized through these experiences in community-based leadership. To many stakeholders, consensus-based decision processes were a new experience, one that promoted a broader understanding of different points of view as well as community ownership of the projects. Experiences with strategic planning, needs assessment, program development, and evaluation also encouraged skill development among the participants. Feedback from community participants further confirmed that the sum total of these resource investments did strengthen the communities' ability to address youth and family issues as well as more generally to work together toward community goals (as is detailed in a later section).

WAS TPPI A SUCCESS AS A TEEN
PREGNANCY PREVENTION EFFORT?

Two separate perspectives can be taken to judge the success of TPPI: (a) as a community-based health promotion project and (b) as a teen pregnancy prevention intervention. Because this initiative was community determined from the beginning, the views of the participants become an initial basis for judging project success. In addition, more objective consideration must be given to whether the accomplishments of this intervention are likely to have long-term impacts on the communities involved.

Although age-specific fertility rates declined in each of the TPPI project areas (with the exception of one age group in one community), the simultaneous reduction in teen childbearing across most areas of the United States limits these downward trends as indicators of the success of TPPI activities. Moreover, few of the program activities funded within the TPPI communities were prolonged or intensive enough to produce community-level changes in age-specific fertility rates. Although some programs have reported success in reducing the second pregnancy rates among their case-managed clients (Grimm, 2000; Wilson & Hagan, 1999), these changes are unlikely to be responsible for overall changes in teen pregnancy rates that have been observed.

Despite these caveats, the presumption underlying all community-based interventions designed to prevent teen pregnancy is that changes in the community setting in which teen pregnancy occurs ultimately will have an effect on the prevalence of this problem. Previous sections have demonstrated a generalized effort to mobilize community awareness of and involvement in teen pregnancy as an issue. To the extent that such commitment can be sustained, it is fair to conclude that the activities within the TPPI communities, when coupled with other societal efforts to reduce teen pregnancy, will in time have the desired effect of reducing the numbers of children born to teen mothers.

How Should the Success of Community-Based Teen Pregnancy Prevention Interventions Be Defined?

What is realistic to expect in terms of the ability of community-based programs to achieve changes in health-related problems? Evaluations of similar types of efforts have suggested that community coalitions might not be able to effect substantial changes in health status in the short term (Howell et al., 1998; Loda, Speizer, Martin, Skatrud, & Bennett, 1997). Other observers have noted that community-based teen pregnancy prevention initiatives differ from more traditional interventions in several key ways:

Many community-level efforts place emphasis on creating greater awareness and understanding of teen pregnancy as a first priority. Helping the community to understand the importance of a problem is the first step toward promoting greater commitment toward solving it. Some criticize community-based coalitions for focusing more on the importance of teen pregnancy than on specific solutions (Loda et al., 1997). Others maintain that promoting awareness is a very pragmatic approach given the controversies surrounding teen pregnancy (Nezlek & Galano, 1993).

Community-level planning tends to gravitate toward short-term outcomes and narrow definitions of the problems (Kreuter & Lezin, 1998; White & Whelage, 1995). Community-based coalitions are typically encouraged to start with "doable" projects that are concrete, attainable, and measurable so as to build momentum and keep member commitment. Ideally, these activities are directly related to the successful functioning of the coalitions as well as working toward the resolution of complex problems such as teen pregnancy (Hancock et al., 1997; Mattessich & Monsey, 1997; Winer & Ray, 1994). The question to be asked is whether the process of engaging the community in an issue such as teen pregnancy has value, irrespective of how effective individual activities may be in reducing the numbers of teens who become pregnant.

The prevention strategies judged by community members to be the most effective are those that relate to youth values and skills, whereas more controversial strategies tend to have less support (Center for the Study of Social Policy, 1995). In general, strategies designed to build on community assets appear to encourage citizen participation to a greater extent than do those that focus on problems or deficiencies (Kingsley, McNeely, & Gibson, 1997; Kretzmann & McKnight, 1993; Winer & Ray, 1994). Finding a noncontroversial middle ground from which to work has been a particular challenge for teen pregnancy prevention efforts. Although most recognize teen pregnancy as a serious problem, there is substantial debate at the community level about how the problem should be approached and about the most effective strategies to be used. Options that tend *not* to be chosen are those that generate controversy such as sex education, contraceptive availability, and school-based clinics (White & Whelage, 1995).

After 5 years of planning and implementing programs to reduce teen pregnancy, stakeholders in the five TPPI communities were asked what else the community should do to reduce teen pregnancy. Their open-ended suggestions indicate that the stakeholders in each of the communities would continue in the same programmatic areas: education, resource development, and increasing community involvement and dialogue.

Various interpretations can be given to the directions in which the programs in the five TPPI grantee communities have developed. At one level, it might be said that the TPPI communities have incorrectly understood the root causes of teen pregnancy and are developing programs that assume that knowledge and awareness alone will lead to change in the numbers of teen pregnancies (White & Whelage, 1995). Another view might be that the stakeholders in the TPPI communities have been pragmatic, adopting strategies that they know can be implemented and that respond to widely recognized community needs. The broadest view, however, is that the strategies adopted within the TPPI communities address a more fundamental issue at the heart of a variety of social problems: the lack of social capital. Social capital has been variously defined to include civic engagement, trust, and willingness to help others in the community. Clear links have been made between health indicators and the levels of social capital in individual communities (Easterling, Gallagher, Drisko, & Johnson, 1998). Less is known, however, about how social capital might be developed.

Social capital begins with relationships among residents, neighborhood institutions, service providers, and public and private funders. From this perspective, a collaborative effort should be judged not only in terms of changes in health status per se but also in terms of the ways in which community ties have been fostered and strengthened. Moreover, efforts to develop social capital ideally should lead to a broader community capacity to deal with a variety of problems.

The data presented in this chapter do not allow us to determine the extent to which levels of social capital increased in the five TPPI communities. A summary of key findings from this report suggests, however, that one of the major accomplishments of TPPI was its ability to encourage communities to enhance their approach to solving problems in ways that in turn will ultimately increase community levels of social capital:

- *Diverse stakeholders* representing various agency perspectives, ideological points of view, and both provider and consumer interests were convened and successfully completed a strategic planning process.
- Throughout the subsequent implementation period, stakeholders played a major role in supporting and providing *community oversight* of the prevention interventions that were put in place.
- The process for decision making, which required ongoing meetings and dialogue, encouraged community ownership of the project and also *promoted networking* among the participants.
- Substantial effort was made to *increase community awareness and involvement* in teen pregnancy prevention issues. Stakeholders have indicated that this was one of the major accomplishments of TPPI.
- The TPPI project directors were able to leverage their program funds to *increase services and resources for families and youth* as well as to engage in other

community-level initiatives to *promote youth-oriented program development.* Increases in services are among the more visible impacts of TPPI.

- The TPPI project directors were able to encourage the development of a broader statewide initiative promoting the *development of youth assets initiatives* in communities throughout Colorado.
- Several of the community-level projects initiated with TPPI support are *likely to continue* through local support supplemented by other funding sources. Examples are the charter school for pregnant and parenting teens in Montrose and the adoption of expanded case management services within Denver Kids in the West Denver community.

Will the dialogue continue? The stakeholders have indicated through their survey that more work remains to be done. An overwhelming majority (94%) indicated that they would participate in a project such as this again. The challenge in continuing this work centers around the difficulties that communities have in obtaining grant funding to continue community development work. Each of the communities has put substantial effort into resource development, only to find that long-term sources of support for programs such as this are hard to identify. Local fund-raising campaigns, program diversification, and joint ventures have been some of the more successful strategies that the TPPI projects have used to continue their program efforts. It is ironic that whether the TPPI programs remain viable may have less to do with their program successes and more to do with the limited sources of funding support to sustain programs of this type.

What Factors Influence the Success Achieved?

From the perspective of participants TPPI was a success in three specific areas: community awareness, resource development, and collaboration/ networking. What factors facilitated these accomplishments?

All in all, the process evaluation results suggest that there were many elements of TPPI that promoted and supported the initiative's overall goals. With 5 years of funding, the *length of TPPI* allowed the project directors to make continuing refinements after learning what worked and what did not work. The *ample funding* ensured that a lack of resources was not a reason for inaction or for a lack of project momentum. Of particular benefit was the presence of a *full-time project director* in each of the communities.

At the same time, the *flexibility* that was allowed to the grantees resulted in projects that were very *individualistic* in all of the grantee communities. The requirement that all *representative* voices be included and that *consensus* be reached tended to narrow down the prevention options considered. As detailed earlier, none of the communities addressed contraceptive availability as a

Table 4.6   Reactions of TPPI Stakeholders to Key Initiative Components

	Number Responding	Percentage "Agreeing" or "Strongly Agreeing"
Group consensus about necessary teen pregnancy programs and services provided a foundation for future program development.	98	80
The flexibility of the planning process promoted community ownership.	97	74
Having money for program implementation allowed community needs to be met.	97	86

NOTE: Only stakeholders participating in the planning process during the first year of TPPI answered the questions concerning this part of the initiative.

	Number Responding	Percentage "Agreeing" or "Strongly Agreeing"
Has TPPI increased community dialogue about teen pregnancy health issues?	162	80
Has TPPI increased people's willingness to work together?	161	78

possible prevention strategy, in part because of the controversy it would be likely to generate and in part because of stakeholder perceptions that making contraceptives available is not as effective a prevention strategy as are other options. Stakeholders, however, have a different view of the consensus requirement. In a 1998 survey, 80% saw the need to reach consensus as necessary to build continuing community support for future teen pregnancy prevention efforts. Stakeholder reactions to other initiative components are provided in the Table 4.6.

Conclusion

TPPI represented a unique experiment in how communities go about dealing with health promotion-type issues. Teen pregnancy prevention is among the most controversial and contentious issues. Key lessons offered by the TPPI experience relate to how communities select and implement activities designed to prevent teen pregnancy, starting from their own perspectives regarding which prevention strategies are deemed to be effective and based on their individual definitions of needs in their communities. This strategy of community engagement is one currently recommended by the National Campaign to Prevent Teen Pregnancy and is also part of the Centers for Disease Control and Prevention's Community Coalition Partnership Program for the Prevention of Teen Pregnancy. The Colorado experience suggests that when community groups use consensus-based decision making to select among teen pregnancy prevention strategies, these groups are less likely to select controversial strategies. At the same time, however, the use of consensus-based decision making creates a basis of ownership that encourages communities to define their projects as successful based on increased community awareness of teen pregnancy, increased development of resources for families and youth, and increased collaboration among local agencies and stakeholders.

Beyond community engagement, the achievements of the five TPPI communities suggest a broader investment in social capital, now recognized as a critical component of overall community health. The future of these efforts remains unclear within the individual TPPI grantee communities, yet the resource base and human capital developed through TPPI funding offer a solid foundation from which future community-based activities can be developed. Time will tell how able the five community projects are to continue the work they have begun.

Note

1. These include the Annie E. Casey Foundation's Plain Talk initiative, the Centers for Disease Control and Prevention's Community Coalition Partnership Program for the Prevention of Teen Pregnancy, and Minnesota's Teen Pregnancy Prevention Initiative.

References

Altman, D., Endres, J., Linzer, J., Howard-Pitney, B., Lorig, K., & Rogers, T. (1991). Obstacles to and future goals of ten comprehensive community health promotion projects. *Journal of Community Health, 16,* 299–314.

Anderson, E. (1991). Neighborhood effects on teenage pregnancy. In C. Jencks & P. E. Peterson (Eds.), *The urban underclass* (pp. 375–398). Washington, DC: Brookings Institution.

Brindis, C. (1992). Adolescent pregnancy prevention for Hispanic youth: The role of schools, families, and communities. *Journal of School Health, 62,* 345–351.

Bruner, C. (1991). *Thinking collaboratively: Ten questions and answers to help policy makers improve children's services.* Washington, DC: Education and Human Services Consortium.

Card, J. J., Brindis, C., Paterson, J. L., &. Niego, S. (1999). *Guidebook: Evaluating teen pregnancy prevention programs.* Los Altos, CA: Sociometrics.

Center for the Study of Social Policy. (1995). *Building new futures for at-risk youth: Findings from a five year multi-site evaluation.* Washington, DC: Author.

Connell, J. P., Kubisch, A. C., Schorr, L. B., & Weiss, C. H. (1995). *New approaches to evaluating community initiatives.* Washington, DC: Aspen Institute.

Connell, J. P., Spencer, M. B., & Aber, J. L. (1994). Educational risk and resiliency in African-American youth: Context, self, action, and outcomes in school. *Child Development, 65,* 493–506.

Dash, L. (1989). *When children want children.* New York: Penguin Books.

Easterling, D., Gallagher, K., Drisko, J., & Johnson, T. (1998). *Promoting health by building community capacity: Evidence and implications for grantmakers.* Denver: The Colorado Trust.

Frost, J. J., & Forrest, J. D. (1995). Understanding the impact of effective teenage pregnancy prevention programs. *Family Planning Perspectives, 27*(5), 188–195.

Gallagher, K., & Drisko, J. (1998). *Stories from the field: Impacts of The Colorado Trust's Teen Pregnancy Prevention 2000 Initiative.* Denver: The Colorado Trust.

Grimm, S. (2000). *Program evaluation compendium, Aurora Teen Pregnancy Prevention Project.* Denver: The Colorado Trust.

Hancock, L., Samson, R. W., Redman, S., Burton, R., Burton, L., Butler, J., Girgis, A., Gibberd, R., Hensley, M., McClintock, A., Reid, A., Schoefield, M., Tripodi, T., & Walsh, R. (1997). Community action for health promotion: A review of methods and outcomes, 1990–1995. *American Journal of Preventive Medicine, 13,* 229–239.

Hayes, C. D. (1987). *Risking the future, adolescent sexuality, pregnancy, and childbearing.* Washington, DC: National Academy Press.

Howard, M., & McCabe, J. (1992). An information and skills approach for younger teens: Postponing Sexual Involvement program. In B. Miller, J. Card, J. Paikoff, & J. Peterson (Eds.), *Preventing adolescent pregnancy: Model programs and evaluations* (pp. 83–109). Newbury Park, CA: Sage.

Howard, M., & Mitchell, M. E. (1993). Preventing teenage pregnancy: Some questions to be answered and some answers to be questioned. *Pediatric Annals, 22*(2), 109–118.

Howell, E. M., Devaney, B., McCormick, M., & Raykovich, K. T. (1998). Back to the future: Community involvement in the Healthy Start program. *Journal of Health, Politics, and Law, 23,* 291–317.

Hutchins, J. (1999). Promising approaches to preventing teen pregnancy. In T. Kreinin, S. Kuhn, A. B. Rodgers, & J. Hutchins (Eds.), *Get organized: A guide to preventing teen pregnancy* (pp. 5–28). Washington, DC: National Campaign to Prevent Teen Pregnancy.

Institute of Medicine. (1995). *The best intentions: Unintended pregnancy and the well-being of children and families.* Washington, DC: National Academy Press.

Kingsley, G. T., McNeely, J. B., & Gibson, J. O. (1997). *Community building: Coming of age.* Washington, DC: Urban Institute.

Kirby, D. (1997). *No easy answers: Research findings on programs to reduce teen pregnancy.* Washington, DC: National Campaign to Prevent Teen Pregnancy.

Kotloff, L. J., Roaf, P. A., & Gambone, M. A. (1995). *The Plain Talk planning year: Mobilizing communities to change.* Philadelphia: Public/Private Ventures.

Kretzmann, J. P., & McKnight, J. L. (1993). *Building communities from the inside out: A path toward finding and mobilizing a community's assets.* Chicago: ACTA Publications.

Kreuter, M., & Lezin, N. (1998). *Are consortia/collaboratives effective in changing health status and health systems? A critical review of the literature.* Report prepared for the Office of Planning, Evaluation, and Legislation, Health Resources and Services Administration, Rockville, MD.

Kreuter, M., Young, L., & Lezin, N. (1998). *Measuring social capital in small communities.* Atlanta, GA: Health 2000.

Lawson, A., & Rhode, D. (1993). *The politics of pregnancy, adolescent sexuality, and public policy.* Port Chester, NY: National Professional Resources.

Loda, F. A., Speizer, I. S., Martin, K. L., Skatrud, J. D., & Bennett, T. A. (1997). Programs and services to prevent pregnancy, childbearing, and poor birth outcomes among adolescents in rural areas of the southeastern United States. *Journal of Adolescent Health, 21,* 57–166.

Luker, K. (1996). *Dubious conceptions: The politics of teenage pregnancy.* Cambridge, MA: Harvard University Press.

Mattessich, P., & Monsey, B. (1997). *Community-building: What makes it work? A review of factors influencing successful community building.* St. Paul, MN: Amherst H. Wilder Foundation.

Miller, B. C., Card, J. J., Paikoff, R. L., & Peterson, J. L. (1992). *Preventing adolescent pregnancy model programs and evaluations.* Newbury Park, CA: Sage.

Minkler, M. (1997). *Community organizing and community building for health.* New Brunswick, NJ: Rutgers University Press.

National Campaign to Prevent Teen Pregnancy. (1998). *While the adults are arguing, the teens are getting pregnant: Overcoming conflict in teen pregnancy prevention.* Washington, DC: Author.

National Campaign to Reduce Teen Pregnancy. (1997). *Whatever happened to childhood? The problem of teen pregnancy in the United States.* Washington, DC: Author.

Nezlek, J. B., & Galano, J. (1993). Developing and maintaining state-wide adolescent pregnancy prevention coalitions: A preliminary investigation. *Health Education Research, Theory, & Practice, 8,* 433–447.

Philiber, S., & Namerow, P. (1995). *Trying to maximize the odds: Using what we know to prevent teen pregnancy* (prepared for the Teen Pregnancy Prevention Program, Division of Reproductive Health). Atlanta, GA: Centers for Disease Control and Prevention.

Price, R. H., Cioci, M., Penner, W., & Trautlein, B. (1993). Webs of influence: School and community programs that enhance adolescent health and education. *Teachers College Record, 94,* 487–521.

Research and Evaluation, Drisko, J., & Gallagher, K. (1995). *Stakeholder attitudes towards teen pregnancy, its causes, and solutions.* Denver: University of Colorado Health Sciences Center, Department of Family Medicine.

Research and Evaluation, Drisko, J., & Gallagher, K. (1997). *Parents talk about raising teens in the 90s.* Denver: University of Colorado Health Sciences Center, Department of Family Medicine.

Scales, P. C., & Leffert, N. (1999). *Developmental assets: A synthesis of the scientific research on adolescent development.* Minneapolis, MN: Search Institute.

Schorr, L. B. (1988). *Within our reach: Breaking the cycle of disadvantage.* New York: Doubleday.

Trussell, J., Card, J. J., & Hogue, C. J. R. (1998). Adolescent sexual behavior, pregnancy, and childbearing. In R. Hatcher (Ed.), *Contraceptive technology.* New York: Irvington.

White, J. A., & Whelage, G. (1995). Community collaboration: If it is such a good idea, why is it so hard to do? *Education Evaluation and Policy Analysis, 17*(1), 23–38.

Wilson, N., & Hagan, N. (1999). *The Colorado Trust's expansion of the initiative to support local evaluation: Delta/Montrose Teen Pregnancy Prevention Initiative.* Denver: The Colorado Trust.

Winer, M., & Ray, K. (1994). *Collaboration handbook: Creating, sustaining, and enjoying the journey.* St. Paul, MN: Amherst H. Wilder Foundation.

Zabin, L. (1992). School-linked reproductive health services: The Johns Hopkins program. In B. Miller, J. Card, J. Paikoff, & J. Peterson (Eds.), *Preventing adolescent pregnancy model programs and evaluations* (pp. 156–184). Newbury Park, CA: Sage.

5

The Community Action for Health Promotion Initiative

Building Capacity in Small, Focused, Community-Based Health Promotion Programs

Douglas H. Fernald

Deborah S. Main

Carolyn J. Tressler

Kathryn A. Judge Nearing

During the past decade, communities have received increased recognition as leaders and participants in promoting the health and well-being of residents, tackling health issues ranging from heart disease to HIV infection to teenage pregnancy. The impacts of the largest, federally funded, community-based health promotion programs have been widely reported, but we continue to know very little about the accomplishments of smaller community-based health promotion programs (e.g., those with annual budgets of $10,000 or less), even though these more modest programs are far more common.

The Community Action for Health Promotion Initiative (CAHPI) was a 5-year, $4.5 million initiative funded by The Colorado Trust to meet the unique health needs of individual communities and to build local capacity for health promotion through community-initiated efforts. The goals of CAHPI were to (a) increase local health promotion activities in Colorado through the development and support of collaborative, community-based projects and (b) enhance the capacity of Colorado communities to identify and address local preventable health problems.

Although many community-based health promotion projects aim to reduce chronic disease using large-scale, statewide, or national programs, CAHPI was designed with the premise that shorter term focused efforts can also have positive effects on health promotion and disease prevention. In particular, it was assumed that by giving communities the predominant role in identifying their critical health issues and in deciding how to address those issues, the resultant programs would be more relevant to the target communities and more likely to be sustained over a longer period of time compared with a more prescribed approach. Moreover, this initiative was purposefully designed to build capacity for health promotion through locally initiated activities, creating a host of efforts to support the health and well-being of citizens across Colorado.

As such, CAHPI provides a unique opportunity to learn more about small, focused, community-based health promotion programs, which are common in communities across Colorado and the nation. This chapter addresses the viability of small health promotion projects as a mechanism for promoting community health. We describe both the strengths and the weaknesses of this approach to community health promotion and elucidate the common challenges faced by these modestly funded programs. Finally, we discuss the implications of our findings in terms of how those who support these efforts (e.g., funding agencies, technical assistance providers) can enhance the capacity of these small health promotion programs to improve the health of people and communities.

Description of the Community Health Promotion Grant Program

Because of its nearly decade-long history in working with Colorado communities around health promotion, Colorado Action for Healthy People (CAHP) was selected by The Colorado Trust to administer and manage the review of proposals and projects, to disburse funds to grantees, and to provide technical assistance.

Through CAHPI, grantees were awarded a maximum of $10,000 per year for up to 3 years and were expected to leverage additional in-kind resources from their communities. Grants were distributed and re-awarded 1 year at a

Table 5.1   Community Grants by Health Issue

Health Issue	Number of Grantees
Nutrition and exercise	11
Adult wellness	8
Adolescent health	7
Childhood injury	6
Violence prevention	5
Healthy habits for children	5
Tobacco use prevention and cessation	4
Heart disease prevention	2

time. Between August 1995 and August 2001, the initiative funded 48 local health promotion projects around Colorado. Although most projects were funded for the full duration allowed under the guidelines of the grants (3 years in most cases), two projects ceased their participation in the initiative after the first year and one project terminated its participation after 2 years. These projects addressed eight distinct areas of health promotion, as shown in Table 5.1.

Each funded project was assigned a program officer from the managing agency who provided primarily telephone-based technical assistance to the project director to guide both the development and the implementation of the project. Each project, in turn, designated its own project director to manage the project at the local level. These project directors had highly variable levels of experience in community health promotion, grant management, and project management. Accordingly, the technical assistance that CAHP provided to these project directors varied substantially.

One of the most unique aspects of CAHPI was that grantees were offered technical assistance even before they were approved for funding. In particular, CAHP provided feedback, guidance, and coaching to applicants during the proposal-writing phase of the process. After this early phase, CAHP offered technical assistance in response to the needs voiced by individual grantees, especially in the areas of budgeting and developing objectives, action steps, and measures. Grantees were also provided referrals to consultants beyond CAHP as well as to other key contacts around the state. One of the most important services that CAHP provided grantees was ongoing support and encouragement throughout the various phases of the project. Most (about 90%) of the one-on-one technical assistance was provided by telephone. Although this assistance covered a variety of topics, CAHP most frequently helped grantees with budget issues, facilitating relationships and communications with others (i.e., networking), and planning program activities.

"Group-level" technical assistance was delivered through grantees meetings—held twice a year for 1 to 1½ days—and covered more general topics such as evaluation, grant writing, objectives writing, and information relevant to the health topics of the convened project directors. These presentations were usually fairly brief, lecture-style presentations with opportunities for some grantee participation. Grantees meetings also offered project directors opportunities for networking and resource sharing.

Description of the Evaluation

The Community Action for Health Promotion Initiative provides an excellent opportunity to learn more about the effect that limited levels of funding and technical support have on a community's capacity to plan and implement health promotion activities at the local level. Through case examples, we designed an evaluation that used a blend of quantitative and qualitative data to generate the following:

- A comprehensive description of the project implementation in CAHPI communities and of the features of the community contexts relevant to each project
- An analysis of the community mobilization process and features of the community contexts that may influence project scope (narrow vs. broad) and sustainability
- An evaluation of the successes, frustrations, challenges, and strategies that constitute the key lessons learned from the projects' experiences.

DATA COLLECTION METHODS

To address these and other evaluation issues, we used several data collection methods, as described in Table 5.2. The core sources of data were in-depth semi-structured interviews with project directors, project progress reports, surveys, and semiannual grantees meetings. Additional sources of data included interviews and discussions with CAHP staff, project proposals and continuation proposals, interviews with other project staff or community members, and site visits where appropriate. We collected most of our data from projects that received grants from the fall of 1995 through the fall of 1998. Less comprehensive data were collected from a fifth cohort of projects funded in the fall of 1999.

The interviews routinely asked respondents to think about project successes, challenges, changes, assistance or resource needs, interactions with CAHP staff, reactions to the project, and thoughts about the project's future. The surveys gathered information about the types of technical assistance received and about the project participants' perceptions of their personal development and working relations with others. When our data collection

Table 5.2   CAHPI Data Collection Grid

Method	Source	Data
Key informant interviews	Project directors, project coordinators, CAHP staff, and other people close to projects	In-depth information about personnel, project activities, community context, and collaborative efforts
Site visits	Project directors or coordinators and others	Community context and data on events and people
Grantees meetings	Project directors or coordinators and guests	Project updates (including successes and challenges) that directors provided at grantees meetings
ET/CAHP meetings	CAHP staff	Updates on individual projects
Incidental contacts with sites	Project directors or coordinators and others	Information on project status, events, and so on
Focused discussion	CAHP staff	Discussion with CAHP staff reflecting on CAHPI in terms of organizational change, learnings, procedural changes, successes, challenges, the future, and stories
Technical assistance survey	Project directors or coordinators	Technical assistance from managing agency or other sources (e.g., frequency, type, source)
Self-assessment survey	Project directors or coordinators	Project director skills and knowledge development from beginning of involvement with CAHPI to end of involvement with CAHPI
Working with others survey	Project directors or coordinators	Assessments of who contributes, how they contribute, how often they contribute, and aspects of the relationship itself (e.g., value, length, impact of grant)

Table 5.2   Continued

Method	Source	Data
6-month progress report summaries	Project directors or coordinators	Reviews and summaries of these reports submitted by projects (as required by grants) with data on accomplishments, barriers, collaboration, volunteers, and community context
Continuation proposal summaries	Project directors or coordinators	Reviews and summaries of the proposals submitted by grantees seeking another year of funding; data on current activities, updates to collaboration, changes in project activities and objectives, and budget information
Original proposals	Project directors or coordinators	Summaries of original proposals submitted by prospective grantees
Document reviews	Usually local media	Summaries of local media, local evaluation data, other local data, or other project or community documents
Community profiles	Census bureau, chambers of commerce, Colorado Department of Labor, Colorado Department of Education, and various county agencies	Short summaries of each community's economic, geographic, demographic, and educational data

NOTE: CAHPI = Community Action for Health Promotion Initiative; CAHP = Colorado Action for Healthy People; ET = Evaluation Team.

ended, we had conducted more than 200 in-depth interviews with project directors and other key informants in the communities or at CAHP and had made more than 50 visits to communities around the state, observing and participating in local projects and activities.

The data were analyzed on an ongoing basis to provide initiative-level feedback and recommendations to The Colorado Trust and CAHP as well as to allow for refinements in the evaluation design. Because most of our data were qualitative, we employed several individual and team approaches to analysis, including reflective "memoing," grounded theory techniques (Denzin & Lincoln, 1994), and "template" and "editing" styles of analysis (Crabtree & Miller, 1999). Such methods generally produce results inductively, such that a researcher starts with a "blank slate" and allows the data to guide the discovery of evolving patterns or themes. Our extensive cross-case analyses drew on all of our data sources to generate learnings that reflect the collective experience, knowledge, wisdom, and advice from those working at the "ground level" on community-based health promotion activities throughout the state.

Although we collected detailed information on a site-by-site basis, the evaluation was designed to describe and characterize the impacts and effects of CAHPI as a whole. Because of the number and diversity of projects (in terms of health focuses, approaches, experiences, and locales), evaluating and reporting on individual projects would have been impractical. Therefore, we worked to generate learnings that could be generalized across individual programs, presenting the overall picture of the course and consequences of the initiative. We collected data to highlight important features of the overall initiative, what did and did not work, and what happened (whether intended or unintended). In considering this global perspective on the initiative, we tried to assess what did and did not happen based on our understanding of the initiative's two goals: (a) to increase locally based health promotion activities and (b) to build the capacity of these communities to identify and address preventable health problems.

The findings presented in what follows are based on the careful analysis of the patterns that emerged from our data, including the hundreds of telephone interviews, surveys, project progress reports, numerous site visits, and grantees meetings attended. We summarize the most salient issues, themes, ideas, factors, and emerging lessons from all of the sites that collectively help to define a community's capacity to carry out important health promotion work, regardless of the particular health issue addressed.

Program Impacts

INCREASED COMMUNITY-BASED HEALTH PROMOTION ACTIVITIES IN COLORADO

Increasing community-based health promotion activities in Colorado was a primary goal of CAHPI. In this section, we provide evidence as to how communities increased the number and scope of health promotion programs and activities in a variety of ways.

CAHPI supported a diversity of organizations, implementation strategies, and target populations. Among the organizations represented in the 48 projects were schools, churches, hospitals, libraries, nursing services, health departments, family resource centers, and community service organizations. The community-based nature of these organizations also varied from strong grassroots groups, to loose networks of organizations, to structured and sophisticated agencies.

As a requirement of the grants, projects were asked to employ multiple strategies to address the chosen health issues. Local projects incorporated an array of intervention strategies for their programs, including the following:

- Education programs aimed at individuals (e.g., students, parents, professionals)
- General education and awareness programs (e.g., posters, educational materials, public service announcements, outreach programs)
- Participatory events or activities (e.g., forums/conferences, community meetings, health fairs, exercise classes, speakers)
- Youth activities (e.g., mentoring programs, after-school programs)
- Health services or products (e.g., counseling, health screenings, reduced-cost or free products such as car seats and child safety kits, resource libraries)
- Community development or capacity-building interventions (e.g., *promotoras* or neighborhood outreach workers, coalitions, planning groups)

The 48 projects targeted their activities toward different populations, ranging from infants to seniors and from neighborhoods to county-based interventions. In the Denver metropolitan area, target populations were generally focused on neighborhoods or particular areas of the city, whereas in more rural or outlying areas of the state, target populations ranged from schools, to entire counties, to multiple counties. Age ranges for target populations covered a spectrum that included infants, school children, adolescents/teens, adults, seniors, and combinations of these. In addition, projects targeted special at-risk populations as relevant to community needs and organizational goals. These populations included African Americans, Latinos, Native Americans, parents, and those at risk for specific illnesses (e.g., osteoporosis, diabetes, cardiovascular disease).

The projects were diverse not only in terms of focus, scope, and strategies but also in terms of their preexisting organizational capacity, defined in terms of existing infrastructure,[1] experienced staff working on the projects, and expertise in the particular health content focuses of the projects. At the time they received funding, about 15% of the funded projects had all three components of capacity: existing infrastructure support, experienced people involved with their projects, and specific expertise in the particular health promotion focuses of the grants. For these projects, the grant funds were typically used to replicate or expand on larger existing programs. About half of the funded projects indicated that they had existing infrastructure and experienced staff. They used the funding to develop and implement programs in new health content areas and to hire staff to implement those programs. The remaining projects reported having some existing infrastructure in place (e.g., a school, a nonprofit organization) but needed the funding to hire new staff *and* to develop new programs that would not otherwise have existed.

Consistent with one of its primary goals, CAHPI resulted in the development or expansion of nearly 50 health promotion programs across the state of Colorado. The evaluation found that these funded projects were able to reach diverse target populations throughout the state using a variety of strategies. The next section describes how the initiative affected the capacity of those individuals who were involved in developing and implementing these community-based health promotion programs.

BUILDING CAPACITY OF COMMUNITIES TO
IDENTIFY AND ADDRESS PREVENTABLE HEALTH PROBLEMS

The second goal of CAHPI was to increase community capacity for designing and implementing health promotion programs. As explained previously, community-based health promotion projects funded by the initiative received a maximum of $10,000 per year for a maximum of 3 years. These diverse projects aspired to enhance a range of outcomes such as increasing physical activity, promoting low-fat eating, facilitating youth resilience to at-risk health behaviors through connection with adult mentors, supporting personal health goals through social activities, and providing health education and other health-related resources. Although there was some overlap across projects in their health-related goals (see Table 5.1), the short duration and modest funding of the grants precluded an examination of long-term health-related outcomes in CAHPI. Instead, the macro-evaluation examined the initiative's impact on *capacity building*. From our viewpoint, capacity building is both a process and a product of community development and health promotion.

The evaluation of CAHPI examined two distinct categories of capacity built by the initiative: (a) leadership and personal growth/development on the part of the project director and (b) collaboration and community mobilization. The next two subsections present results specific to these two areas of capacity.

Leadership/Project Director Growth and Development

Professional growth and personal development among the CAHPI project directors provide perhaps the most specific examples of how the initiative increased community capacity. In many communities, CAHPI developed new leaders who would continue to develop their skills and capacities in community-based health promotion after the initiative ended. For many project directors, CAHPI served as a "training ground" for learning the knowledge and skills required to develop and implement community projects, whereas for others, the initiative provided the opportunity to continue the community or health promotion work they had been doing for years (Fawcett et al., 1995; Freudenberg et al., 1995; Goodman, Steckler, Hoover, & Schwartz, 1993).

Our assessment of changes in leadership and individual-level capacity focused on the following factors that have been found to be important to the success of small health promotion grants: knowledge and skills about community organizing, communication, leveraging resources, and understanding group process. These skills are relevant to carrying out effective health promotion programs.

By assessing self-reported knowledge and skills of project directors at the beginning and end of their involvement in CAHPI, the evaluation demonstrated changes in knowledge, confidence, and skills developed over the projects' lives, particularly among those who began their directorships with the least experience. Table 5.3 summarizes changes in the capacity of project directors involved in CAHPI along a number of dimensions. This table shows the magnitude of change in the knowledge and skills of project directors who had either no experience or little, moderate, or high levels of experience when they became involved in the initiative. It is important to note that the table highlights data on changes within—not between—project directors with different levels of experience.

In interviews as well, project directors were clear that they had gained knowledge and experience through their participation in their CAHPI projects. One project director described the knowledge gained in two areas: "I have learned about our target population and the challenges in evaluating them." Another added, "I've expanded my thoughts on how to look at our topic. Whether it is evaluating a program or managing a budget, I've been given new ways to approach the situation." One project director described the experience she had gained as follows: "Much of this specific project I learned on the job because I inherited the grant when I began work here. I had done some grant writing but got lots of practice with this [CAHPI] grant." Still another project director pointed out one particular area of improvement: "[The project] has made me a better detail person. I'm more the visionary. I like to develop an idea and get people involved, but I hate all the nitty-gritty . . . and there was a lot of nitty-gritty in this project. I buckled under and did it. So I feel more certain that I can do that."

At the beginning of CAHPI, members of the least experienced group of project directors rated themselves with lower levels of skills and knowledge than did those in the most experienced group. This between-group difference

Table 5.3   Project Director Self-Reported Skills and Knowledge Change

Project Director Confidence in Their:	Less Experienced		Moderately Experienced		More Experienced	
	Start of CAHPI[a]	End of CAHPI[b]	Start of CAHPI	End of CAHPI	Start of CAHPI	End of CAHPI
Knowledge about health issue	3.91	7.04	6.38	7.50	7.02	7.68
Ability to carry out project activities	4.44	6.64	6.66	8.46	7.73	8.07
Ability to carry out grant-related activities	3.70	7.48	5.80	8.32	7.39	8.50
Ability to involve people and community organizations	3.68	6.74	6.29	7.33	7.26	8.14
Ability to advocate for projects and health issues	3.85	5.38	5.78	7.00	7.06	8.43
Ability to evaluate program	4.12	5.79	5.05	7.25	6.67	7.60

NOTE: Self-reported scales range from 1 to 10. CAHPI = Community Action for Health Promotion Initiative.
a. Sample of 51 project directors surveyed at beginning of CAHPI.
b. Subset of 16 project directors who completed survey after all 3 years in CAHPI.

was substantial across all of the dimensions we measured. Over the course of the initiative, however, those in the least experienced group improved their skills and knowledge to a much greater degree than did members of the most experienced group. By the end of the initiative, the least experienced group had largely "caught up" with the most experienced group.

As for CAHPI's objective to enhance capacity, the initiative was very successful with regard to the least experienced project directors but only somewhat successful with regard to the most experienced project directors. To some extent, this differential level of capacity building reflects a "ceiling" effect; members of the most experienced group started out so high that they simply had less room to grow than did those in the least experienced group. However, for two of the dimensions—general knowledge about health issues and program evaluation—even the most experienced group started out with only moderate levels of capacity. By the end of the initiative, all groups still had room to grow.

This pattern of results has important implications for organizations that fund community-based programs and for groups that provide technical assistance. If a funder wishes to build capacity through *small* grants, greater effects can be obtained by focusing on projects that are relatively new and/or have inexperienced program staff. If a funder is interested in substantially building capacity among more experienced projects and staff, it will be necessary to offer technical assistance that is more intensive or tailored than what was provided under CAHPI.

Building Collaboration and Community Mobilization

In line with its capacity-building objectives, CAHP (1996) stressed the importance of collaboration in strengthening community capacity:

> Community capacity refers to a community's level of available resources, its ability to catalyze community involvement, and its ownership of a health problem and its solutions. Collaboration among different segments of the community is considered essential to building community capacity. (p. 2)

CAHP also required grantees to provide evidence of their collaborative efforts in terms of the numbers of agencies working with the grantees toward common community health promotion goals.

In addition to leadership development (described in the previous subsection), mobilizing segments of a community can be viewed as another critical component of enhancing a community's capacity for health promotion program development (Goodman, 1998; Goodman, Wandersman, Chinman, Imm, & Morrisey, 1996; Kreuter, Lezin, & Young, 2000). Collaborative capacity (or the extent to which others were involved) varied across projects but became an important intermediate step to meeting (or not meeting) project goals and objectives and to sustaining individual health promotion efforts. Data collected during the evaluation confirm that one of the clear impacts of the CAHPI grants was that they fostered new relationships, or strengthened existing relationships, between projects and local collaborative partners. Across the diverse projects undertaken, the number of individuals, organizations, agencies, and businesses that contributed to a project often exceeded the number of collaborators noted in proposals. Through surveys, we collected contributor data from all projects funded during the first three funding cycles. Of the 25 sites reporting, 72% fostered relationships with new contributors during their involvement in CAHPI. All sites reported new or strengthened relationships with at least one contributor where a relationship already existed. The average number of *active* contributors per project was 11, ranging from 3 to 28. Of the 304 active contributors reported by the projects, having a CAHPI grant enabled grantees to strengthen relationships among 38% of their contributors or to sustain existing relationships among 31% of their contributors. Among all of the projects, 26% of the contributors were new to organizations.

Some of the overall findings about working with others, however, suggest additional facets of collaboration within these small grant projects:

- All projects reported that they had developed new or stronger relationships with their active contributors.
- Fully 61% of the active contributors to CAHPI projects were either individuals or organizations with whom project directors had worked only infrequently or not at all prior to the initiative. Thus, involvement in the projects brought new or improved relationships with collaborators and other contributors.

Generating, maintaining, and improving resources outside of the projects was one of the important—albeit sometimes transparent—successes of these small, focused health promotion projects.

Challenges to Promoting Health
With Small, Community-Based Projects

Designing and implementing high-quality health promotion and disease prevention interventions is difficult even under ideal conditions, and it is even more so within the context of community settings. In this section, we briefly describe factors that influenced whether and how CAHPI projects implemented their programs in the manner and quality they intended. These findings were based on more than 200 interviews with project directors and key project staff.

IMPLEMENTING MULTIPLE
STRATEGIES AT MULTIPLE LEVELS

In their initial proposals, the CAHPI grantees proposed locally tailored interventions that relied on multiple strategies and targeted multiple "levels" of the communities (defined subpopulations and settings). Despite the fact that research has clearly demonstrated the value of these more ecological, multilevel approaches to community health promotion (McLeroy, Bibeau, Steckler, & Glanz, 1988; Stokols, 1996), many projects experienced difficulties in implementing these more expansive interventions with their modest funding and relatively short project time lines due to slow project start-up, demands of project-related tasks such as program planning and building collaborations, and generally projects being stretched "too thin." Consequently, some projects narrowed their scope by focusing interventions at only one level or on a single target population. In one project, activities were aimed at bicycle helmet use and car seat safety, requiring two different knowledge bases and implementation approaches. After the first year, the project coordinator and director trimmed the focus to car seat safety only.

DIFFICULTY IN REACHING TARGET POPULATIONS

Among the greatest challenges in implementing health promotion programs is reaching sufficient numbers of the proposed target population(s). The CAHPI projects that proposed to work with more than one target group (e.g., elementary school *and* high school students) often learned that each required a different strategy, demanding different interventions and strategies to increase program participation. Given limited time and project resources, these project efforts often had to be refined over time. Many project directors commented on how they had initially overestimated the interest and willingness of target groups to participate in their health promotion programs. Although some learned to be creative in attracting program participants, others acknowledged that building a stable group of participants would be a much more gradual process that would occur only as they were able to find time to get the word out about their programs.

UNREALISTIC PROGRAM OBJECTIVES AND TIME LINES

Project directors and other key staff most frequently mentioned unrealistic expectations and time lines when explaining their lack of full program implementation. Many said that they did not realize it would take as long as it did to meet their project goals. Some attributed this to a lack of experience, whereas others attributed it to the considerable time it took to get cooperation and buy-in from key staff, volunteers, and program participants. One project director put it this way:

> Don't try to bite off more than you can chew. I tried to pack more in than we could do effectively. It backfired on me. There was a sense of stress and dissatisfaction among the students when they felt rushed. They felt they weren't able to do things in a quality way that they had imagined.

Likewise, another project director said,

> It seems like it should have been a 5-year funding commitment instead of 3 [years]. It takes 3 years to get things off the ground, and that's working really hard at it.

Others agreed that the first year of a project is spent building relationships, initiating the program, learning what is and is not working, and then making changes:

I think we struggled through the [first] year . . . with trying to get everything coordinated. And it was so hard to do it after school and try to keep the number of kids and keep them consistently coming.

TURNOVER

Throughout CAHPI, we observed frequent turnover of key project staff (especially among the project directors or coordinators) and documented the turnover of 35 project directors or coordinators in 18 projects over the course of the initiative. Turnover struck all types of projects and at all phases of projects; it pervaded the initiative. Reasons for staff departures varied and included new jobs, families moving from the area, personal reasons, internal conflict or disagreement, lack of funding, and viewing the director/coordinator position as temporary or interim. Regardless, project directors found turnover to be disruptive, as noted in the following comments from two project directors:

In the beginning, we had more volunteers than we do now. . . . After they left, it was like starting from ground zero.

Any time you hire a new person [in] any organization, it changes everybody else's relationship with everybody else. It's a new dynamic. It has to be managed. And what if the new person, they do something that offends somebody else? . . . And I had to have my antenna out and be aware of all this stuff and deal with it.

Other factors contributing to turnover included insufficient funding for the position, inconsistent vision, mismatched talents to the job, and poor fit with other organizational goals. Data from interviews and surveys from project directors and key staff helped to explain some of the challenges of staff turnover. With the possibility of paying a person a maximum of $10,000 in any given year, it proved difficult to recruit and keep individuals (even on a part-time basis) who have limited or no other sources of funding. Two project directors added the following advice:

I don't know why they have $10,000 as a ceiling, but I think . . ., well, it's good they are putting resources where they are badly needed . . ., but it tends to not be enough. . . . If they were able to provide more money, I think that they would make an impact a lot sooner. . . . Usually an organization cannot take on these kinds of projects without hiring somebody. . . . In poor communities, it's hard for an organization to find someone sitting around who can do this. So you have to hire somebody. . . . And you can't hire someone who can work enough hours to do the job that needs to be done.

It takes staff to get things done. I don't know why this escapes people's understanding. When you talk about making behavior change, you're talking about asking people to eat right, to exercise. You need to have professional people that know what they're doing. And professional people . . . don't volunteer their time. That's why they went to school and learned all those things. They need to make a living. So I think there should be more of an understanding of the resources that I need to get the kind of professional help that I need to get things done.

These results suggest that the requirements of CAHPI would have been more easily met if the funding had been sufficient to hire a person dedicated to seeing the project through on a consistent basis. Although volunteers and collaborators can help, they cannot substitute for regular staff (Kegler, Steckler, McLeroy, & Malek, 1998).

CHANGING FOR PROGRAM
IMPROVEMENT AND SUSTAINABILITY

Interviews of key project staff served as a critical source of information for understanding how proposed projects unfolded in CAHPI communities. In many cases, projects did not implement what they proposed because they identified more appropriate ways in which to accomplish their objectives. This frequently occurred during the first year of grants.

The proposed projects and their components continued to evolve throughout the projects' 3 years, being refined to meet more realistic project goals, to respond to community needs and interests, and to target activities more likely to be sustained. Many programs became more effective when they changed mid-course—by increasing their fit to the needs and values of the communities, project staff, and target populations. One project director commented,

Don't be afraid to change. If something is not working, don't be afraid to try something else and to keep trying it until you find something that is going to work. If we'd tried to do what we'd done the first year, we'd have still been struggling.

Because CAHPI projects and their funding lasted for 3 years, many projects quickly determined which program components would last and which would not, tending to spend more of their time and project resources on those activities that had a greater chance of being sustained. This led to fewer program components being implemented but a higher sustainability among some projects or particular components.

THE VITAL DIFFICULT WORK
IN BUILDING COLLABORATIONS

Project directors were clear that collaboration-building activities take a great deal of time, skill, and resources. They recommended that the most direct way in which a funder could help a grantee develop collaborative resources would be to provide modest increases in staff funding to underwrite the vital function of reaching out to new and existing contributors and collaborators. This increased collaboration, in turn, could help to promote the project's sustainability.

At least one project director pointed out the dilemma of small amounts of funding in these CAHPI projects:

> Understand that with $10,000 you're asking most people to develop and implement at the same time. And that's a lot. You're asking a lot to do with a little, and that takes a person. Somebody has to really give of their time to do it. And so realistically, $10,000 would probably just not even pay for someone's salary. And that's $10,000 and you're asking for 15 to 20 hours a week, and when you're trying to develop and implement, that's not realistic either because start-up programs take so much more.

Another experienced project director noted the lack of skills in other project directors and the need to offer assistance:

> [The grantees] didn't realize how little they knew about just working with others, talking to people, convening meetings, things like that. Having a productive meeting—I'd say that that really wasn't brought in. . . . I just think that would be a good starting point.

Another project director noted,

> Day in, day out, you have to keep at it. Keep doing it, keep plugging. . . . Keep getting people involved. Call them back, get things going, call people, call people, call people. Personal contact.

Both the literature and the project directors underscore the importance of promoting collaboration (Kreuter et al., 2000), yet project directors consistently told us that it takes time to get a project up and running. One said,

> As a result of having many collaborators, it is time-consuming to continually "check in" with them and keep them involved. The contributions of our collaborators have been invaluable.

Among the more experienced project directors, we heard valuable advice for working with contributors, especially volunteers. For example, three project directors offered the following insights:

> A lot of folks have resources but don't always know how to use them or where. So our responsibility is kind of to help them see their niche, and without it being

complicated or fearful. And being sensitive. And also giving them leeway, where they don't feel overwhelmed.

You know, you can't just say, "Oh good, you're a volunteer. You can take charge of all this stuff." You know, they're not going to want to do that. But if they felt that they're a real valuable part of the greater scheme, that with other people who are actually in charge, it makes it easier for them to be involved because they're not overwhelmed.

I always give credit away. I really try when I'm working with volunteers to make sure they get acknowledged, and any students that work with me, I give them letters that acknowledge [their contributions], that can be used for college applications. So there's some payoffs for them.

Although working with others is a requirement of the grants, according to several experienced project directors, this is an overlooked and underfunded area of health promotion projects.

Implications and Recommendations for Implementing Effective Community-Based Health Promotion Programs

This evaluation of CAHPI has helped to uncover the realistic indicators of success and key challenges for small community-based health promotion programs. In CAHPI, projects were funded for a maximum of $10,000 per year for up to 3 years. Because of this relatively short funding period and modest amount of funding to communities, measurable changes in *community-level* health outcomes may be unrealistic. Nonetheless, these small health promotion projects were found to enhance the project management and leadership skills of many project directors.

This section reviews our overall evaluation findings and places them in the context of CAHPI itself as well as the broader field of community-based health promotion. We consider the lessons learned from this initiative that focused broadly on implementing community-based health promotion projects, the community capacity subsequently developed, and the broader implications of the initiative in terms of how communities work to address preventable health problems.

LEADERSHIP/PERSONAL GROWTH AND DEVELOPMENT

CAHPI provided individuals in communities across Colorado with an opportunity to try something with which they may have had little or no previous experience. The initiative clearly resulted in improved skills and capacities among the participants. The least experienced project directors, in particular, reported gains in virtually all areas related to project and grants management, program development, and implementation. As the less experienced project directors developed more skills and confidence, some began to feel more comfortable in trying new things, creating and strengthening collaboration, and expanding their scope of work.

Many of the more experienced project directors consciously nurtured and developed those around them by providing opportunities to develop project-related skills and knowledge through meaningful involvement. Opportunities to become meaningfully involved in the life of a project seemed to enhance the sense of project ownership and enthusiasm among other staff and volunteers. By design, the managing agency did not have a direct role in the selection of project leadership, but the evaluation data from interviews, surveys, and site visits highlight the important role that leadership plays in the design, implementation, and further capacity building of local projects. Strong technical assistance in leadership development and specific, intensive, project-related training can accelerate the acquisition of skills and knowledge that, in turn, can enhance project implementation.

MOBILIZING OTHERS FOR PROJECT SUCCESS

Project directors were both remarkable and relentless in their ability to mobilize people and resources within their communities—a critical piece of capacity building in communities. Project directors told us that this was vital but hard work. Most funded projects were able to generate impressive amounts of in-kind contributions to leverage the grant funding. In some cases, this level of support has been sustained, allowing project efforts to continue beyond CAHPI funding.

Furthermore, we found that the scope and extent of collaboration varied from project to project as well as within projects. Projects were challenged by how to involve others in a meaningful way, especially with regard to recruiting and maintaining volunteers. Identifying and securing the "optimal" contributors (i.e., those who are passionate about the project mission and with whom projects can establish mutually supportive relationships) can accelerate project implementation, but this often requires a great deal of time.

In the areas of collaboration and mobilization, capacity varied across the projects and was developed to a limited extent through technical assistance. Project directors can benefit from training in working with volunteers, developing collaborative relationships, and increased funding specifically dedicated to developing collaborative relationships. As one director put it,

> What's realistic to expect is that partnerships and collaborations should be built. It should not be just a grant. So there needs to be support. And some of the efforts need to go towards that.

TURNOVER

Turnover among project staff and volunteers was common among CAHPI projects. Several project directors suggested that this was due in part to insufficient funding for retaining vital staff. As one observed,

> For me recently, I've felt more turnover. So I always feel like I'm starting over, just when I've brought on someone. And they're learning it. Or I think they've got [it]. Then they need to move on. And they need to move on because they need more money. They've got to move on, and that just continues to be a disappointment.

Although not all turnover can be solved with money, funders should consider levels of funding that are sufficient to hire or retain skilled and knowledgeable staff who can sustain projects, especially at the outset of new projects where new skills or knowledge may be needed.

Summary and Conclusion

Although the literature on community-based health promotion often focuses on the promise and pitfalls of large, well-funded programs, the current analysis has described what happens in much smaller efforts. Interestingly, these evaluation findings both support the results of previous literature and extend our learning on how small, focused health promotion programs can increase community-based health promotion activity and build the capacity of key people involved in these efforts.

We learned that, similar to the case with more highly funded, long-term, community-based health promotion programs, CAHPI project directors faced many challenges in (a) designing and implementing realistic yet effective programs, (b) working within environments that were resource rich yet cash poor, (c) mobilizing and maintaining community volunteers, and (d) building the necessary infrastructure and community support to enhance program sustainability.

Unlike many large initiatives that focused on single health issues or used common approaches for their interventions, CAHPI projects were noteworthy in terms of their differences rather than their commonalties. That is, these small health promotion projects implemented a wide variety of interventions targeting many different populations in a variety of settings. This made the evaluation quite challenging in terms of our ability to derive general observations from what on the surface appeared to be "apples and oranges."

We found several common patterns across these community programs. First, despite receiving only $10,000 per year in a 3-year grant cycle, these community health promotion projects increased health promotion programs for a variety of individuals and groups within the communities. Many projects used strategies geared toward individual change; few implemented environmental-level strategies for change (e.g., policy change). A large percentage of projects were implemented within local health departments. Others tended to be affiliated with smaller nonprofit organizations, with a few designed by members of the community at large.

CAHPI funding gave some grantees the opportunity to try something new or to add something new to existing programs. For other projects, the CAHPI funds provided some additional funds to support what the organization was already planning to do. The more experienced project directors were more realistic (at the outset) in appreciating that the amount of the grants and duration of funding were not sufficient to accomplish a multilevel health promotion project. They knew that they had to leverage existing resources to make this work more manageable. Relatively less experienced project directors soon realized how challenging this work really is.

Some project directors believed that they were just getting going when the funding through CAHPI ended. Some emphasized how organized they had to be to get project planning and implementation far enough along so that sustainability could be possible by the third and final year. In discussing the amount of the CAHPI grants, a few project directors expressed frustration that perhaps there was a lack of understanding about what it takes to implement these types of projects. Other project directors attributed their inability to implement their programs fully to their inexperience. The relatively small amount of funding did have the intended effect of building capacity in the sense that it instilled confidence and motivated projects to go after additional financial support, materials, personnel, and volunteers.

More than anything, CAHPI provided project directors with the opportunity to build personal skills and community support in the area of health promotion. Without the initiative, this capacity building would not have occurred. This is a realistic and important outcome for all community-based health promotion programs. As stated by Mittelmark and colleagues in a review of large, community-based, cardiovascular prevention programs:

> The enduring lesson from exemplar programs is that the core of a successful program is the community organization process. Practical outcomes of [this process] are many: the identification of key community leaders; the activation of those leaders on behalf of the project; the stimulation of citizens and organizations to volunteer time and offer resources; [and] the adoption of prevention as a theme in the workplace, in schools, and in churches. (Mittelmark, Hunt, Heath, & Schmid, 1993), pp. 455–456.

CAHPI promoted those outcomes by helping project directors and other key staff to learn how to implement an effective community organization process in their communities—an important and realistic indicator of success.

Note

1. Infrastructure is defined in terms of existing programs, resources, and missions congruent with proposed health promotion programs. Often such infrastructure increases project access to additional people and resources that would not otherwise be affordable within the budgetary constraints of many small health promotion projects.

References

Colorado Action for Healthy People. (1996, January). Colorado Action for Healthy People issues request for proposals. *Exchange,* pp. 1–2. (Colorado Action for Healthy People)

Crabtree, B. F., & Miller, W. L. (Eds.). (1999). *Doing qualitative research* (2nd ed.). Thousand Oaks, CA: Sage.

Denzin, N. K., & Lincoln, Y. S. (Eds.). (1994). *Handbook of qualitative research.* Thousand Oaks, CA: Sage.

Fawcett, S. B., Paine-Andrews, A., Francisco, V. T., Schultz, J. A., Richter, K. P., Lewis, R. K., Williams, E. L., Harris, K. J., Berkley, J. Y., Fisher, J. L., & Lopez, C M. (1995). Using empowerment theory in collaborative partnerships for community health and development. *American Journal of Community Psychology, 23,* 677–697.

Freudenberg, N., Eng, E., Flay, B., Parcel, G., Rogers, T., & Wallerstein, N. (1995). Strengthening individual and community capacity to prevent disease and promote health: In search of relevant theories and principles. *Health Education Quarterly, 22,* 290–306.

Goodman, R. M. (1998). Principles and tools for evaluating community-based prevention and health promotion programs. *Journal of Public Health Management and Practice, 4*(2), 37–47.

Goodman, R. M., Steckler, A., Hoover, S., & Schwartz, R. (1993). A critique of contemporary community health promotion approaches: Based on a qualitative review of six programs in Maine. *American Journal of Health Promotion, 7,* 208–220.

Goodman, R. M., Wandersman, A., Chinman, M., Imm, P., & Morrisey, E. (1996). An ecological assessment of community-based interventions for prevention and health promotion: Approaches to measuring community coalitions. *American Journal of Community Psychology, 24,* 33–61.

Kegler, M. C., Steckler, A., McLeroy, K., & Malek, S. H. (1998). Factors that contribute to effective community health promotion coalitions: A study of 10 project ASSIST coalitions in North Carolina. *Health Education and Behavior, 25,* 338–353.

Kreuter, M. W., Lezin, N. A., & Young, L. A. (2000). Evaluating community-based collaborative mechanisms: Implications for practitioners. *Health Promotion Practice, 1*(1), 49–63.

McLeroy, K. R.,. Bibeau, D., Steckler, A., &. Glanz, K. (1988). An ecological perspective on health promotion programs. *Health Education Quarterly, 15,* 351–377.

Mittelmark, M. B., Hunt, M. K., Heath, G. W., & Schmid, T. L. (1993). Realistic outcomes: Lessons from community-based research and demonstration programs for the prevention of cardiovascular diseases. *Journal of Public Health Policy, 14,* 437–462.

Stokols, D. (1996). Translating social ecological theory into guidelines for community health promotion. *American Journal of Health Promotion, 10,* 282–298.

6

The Volunteers for Rural Seniors Initiative

Leveraging Community Resources to Meet the Needs of Seniors

Dora G. Lodwick

Allan Wallis

A growing gap exists between the needs of rural seniors and the services available to them. More seniors are choosing to retire in rural communities or to "age in place" there. At the same time, traditional providers of care—family members and neighbors—are less available because of increasing work demands along with the out-migration of younger people. How can the needs of rural seniors be met? More specifically, how can communities assist in meeting some of their basic needs so that the seniors are able to remain as independent residents in their own homes for as long as possible? Finally, can community-based organizations mobilize resources to heighten awareness of, and generate resources to address, an issue frequently invisible to the community?

Community-based efforts develop when communities identify a problem, mobilize resources, and develop strategies for solving the problem (Minkler, 1997). Often community-based organizations are the initiating force in identifying problem areas and in stimulating communities to acknowledge the need and provide the resources necessary to address the problem. Often external resources, including grants, assist the community-based organizations in this work.

The Volunteers for Rural Seniors Initiative (VRSI), funded by The Colorado Trust between 1995 and 2000, performed this function. VRSI encouraged community-based organizations to bridge the gap between senior needs and senior services by distributing grant dollars totaling $1.75 million. The underlying assumption of the initiative was that small grants could provide sufficient incentive for local community organizations to initiate or expand volunteer-based programs that provide services to rural seniors, thereby encouraging communities to address their aging populations.

Over the life of VRSI, 35 grants were awarded with 34 completed. These grants, averaging $15,500 per year over a 3-year period, stimulated the development of new programs and the expansion of existing services. Through VRSI grants, approximately 2,000 volunteers provided an annual average of about 110,000 hours of service to more than 3,700 rural seniors. An evaluation of the program demonstrates that although the services provided were modest, ranging from delivery of meals to assistance with basic home maintenance, they improved the quality of life of seniors and aided in maintaining their independence. Nonetheless, the types and intensity of services provided were not sufficient to assist most people who were experiencing a major health crisis such as a broken hip or significant home maintenance problems.

Context

During the decade of the 1990s, Colorado's population grew by more than 20%. Many rural communities experienced rapid growth during this period while others declined, but virtually all saw an increase in the size of their senior populations. The ranks of seniors in the more rapidly growing rural communities were fed by newcomers seeking a rural setting in which to retire, by former residents returning to towns where they once lived, and by residents aging in place. Even in areas experiencing an overall decline in population, the senior population grew through increased longevity and aging in place. In addition, in declining communities, the proportion of the population comprised of seniors increased as a result of the out-migration of young adults seeking better employment opportunities elsewhere.

This increase of seniors during the 1990s created new challenges for rural Colorado communities as the gap widened between the needs of rural seniors for services and the capacity of formal and informal support systems to provide for them.

When viewed from the perspective of service availability, small towns are hard-pressed to meet the needs of their seniors. Traditionally, family, friends, and neighbors informally helped seniors, allowing them to maintain their independence and to continue living at home. However, this source of support is disappearing as both adult members of households find that they have to work and as teenagers have less time and inclination to provide services such as mowing lawns and doing errands for others.

Small towns also tend to have a limited range of housing options. Seniors who continue to live in the homes where they raised their families often have more space and greater maintenance demands than they can handle. At the same time, they find it difficult to relocate to more appropriate quarters in their own communities. Supported housing alternatives are either extremely limited or not available. Likewise, there is a dearth of support services ranging from public transportation to home care. In short, rural communities may be quiet attractive places in which to retire, but they tend to have limited supports for their senior populations as they grow frail.

In terms of seniors who are seeking services, life in small towns has also been undergoing significant changes. Many of the elderly who are now retiring to rural communities have spent much of their adult lives in urban areas. These seniors have different expectations regarding giving and receiving services. A nurse in a community on Colorado's high plains described the shift in the following way:

> There are people from Denver and Colorado Springs who want to live in the mountains and expect to have services here. The other day I couldn't make a phone call out for 5 hours because all the circuits were busy. . . . Old ranching people are dying off, and not a lot of new ranchers are coming in. For example, an owner of 30,000 acres dies, so the family sells it to a corporate entity that gets a 40-year-old manager. Our clients in the future will buy the land, build a home over 4 to 5 years, and then become snowbirds.[1]

In effect, two distinct populations of seniors are emerging in rural areas: *newcomers* and *old-timers*. The newcomers have weaker informal helping networks but fewer reservations about using formalized services. The second population consists of traditional old-timers who rely on their families, friends, and neighbors for assistance but who are hesitant to seek formal services if their traditional sources of support are not available. These old-timers include people who have lived in the community continuously and those who lived outside of town but have now moved back following the sale of their farms or the death of their spouses. It also includes seniors who once lived in the town, moved away, and have now returned in retirement.

Seniors who are newcomers from urban areas are less likely to have long-standing friends in the community. In addition, service providers describe the difficulties that newcomers have in being accepted into a community. A hospital administrator in a frontier community (with fewer than 50 people per square mile) reported that newcomers, including seniors, were slow to be accepted into the community unless they had family already living there.[2] Cultural differences between the two groups of seniors are significant. As the administrator observed,

> The newcomers are retirees from the Denver area, Nebraska, wherever. They're retirees with independent incomes. . . . [On the other hand, the old-timers are] farmers and ranchers. They're still very independent people. They've been ranchers all their lives . . ., [yet] they can't live anymore out on the ranches because they can't take care of machinery anymore and they can't shovel the snow anymore.[3]

Newcomers who do not have family members living in the same community are more likely to move closer to their adult children when they have a crisis such as breaking a hip or dealing with a major illness. They are also more likely to move away from their new community when they need supportive services that they cannot find there such as assisted living accommodations.

As seniors get frail, the reasons why they leave their homes are very similar across Colorado and the country. Over time, many seniors begin to have episodic difficulties that make them increasingly dependent on family and friends for medical and other types of assistance.[4] As these problems persist, annual visits to children or other relatives become longer until the seniors no longer return home.[5]

In contrast, traditional old-timers who have lived in a rural community for decades are less likely to move away, even when faced with challenging health problems or failing home maintenance. As one rural service provider observed, these seniors end up dying in place:

> People who tend to be here 30 years, they reach 60 [years of age] and they say, "I'm staying. I'm not leaving. I have lived here 30 years, and I ain't leaving home. I don't care what my kids say."[6]

When an old-timer's home falls into disrepair and there is no one available to maintain it, the old-timer is more likely to simply move into a smaller section of the home than to leave. Old-timers' pride of independence also diminishes their willingness to either seek or accept the help of others. One service provider described an individual, who eventually became a client, as being so hostile to outsiders that he would threaten them with a gun as they approached his house. Although that behavior is an extreme example, the intense independence is not.

The changes evident in rural areas of Colorado during the 1990s are likely to continue, and even to accelerate, during the new century. Rural communities are being challenged to accommodate the emerging and ever-changing needs of their senior populations.

The Initiative

In an effort to fill the gap between the needs of seniors and the available services, volunteers are being recruited in many communities. Seniors themselves are being encouraged to become volunteers to improve their quality of life as well as to provide for the needs of others. Similarly, youth have been encouraged or required to volunteer.[7] Encouraging service opportunities among youth expands the pool of volunteers, introduces youth to the idea of giving service, and connects young and old in communities where generations can be separated and suspicious of one another.

Volunteerism presents challenges in rural areas where increasing newcomers bring different expectations about appropriate ways to help. Wilson and Musick (1997) clarify the differences between volunteering and helping:

> Volunteer work is unpaid work provided to parties to whom the worker owes no contractual, familial, or friendship obligations. Formal volunteering is typically carried out in the context of organizations. . . . Helping is more private, volunteering more public; helping is more casual, volunteering more organized. (p. 701)

Helping is usually done within family and friends networks, although more frequently by family members in both rural and urban areas. Women engage in helping more often than do men. In addition, giving help declines with age, particularly in urban areas, primarily because relatives are no longer nearby (Amato, 1993).

Volunteering, in contrast, is closely related to higher education, income, and religiosity. In addition, both men and women are volunteers (Freedman, 1997). Volunteerism is more typical among seniors who are newcomers as opposed to old-timers.

Although engaging the services of volunteers seems like an obvious way in which to provide needed services to seniors, finding, training, and maintaining an adequate pool of volunteers is a daunting task. Rural communities may have strong traditions of helping, but such support is typically offered by people who know one another. Extending the ethic of volunteering through more formal channels and to "strangers" presents an additional challenge. Finding adequate volunteer resources also means that the pool of volunteers serving seniors must be enlarged without taking them away from organizations that are already using them to provide other services.

The Volunteers for Rural Seniors Initiative encouraged community-based organizations to define community needs related to seniors. The organizations then stimulated the development of volunteers, a community resource, to meet the needs of seniors. It was hoped that the actions of the community-based programs would stimulate the broader community to acknowledge the senior service needs and sustain the programs, thereby filling the gap between limited services and senior needs.

VRSI GOALS AND SCOPE

The overall size of VRSI, $1.75 million to be expended, was regarded as modest by The Colorado Trust's standards. Consequently, the initiative was expected to achieve relatively modest impacts. The objective was to support community-based organizations already using volunteers to serve seniors, to encourage program expansion (providing additional services or expanding service areas), and to motivate organizations not already providing services to seniors to initiate new programs. Organization building was only minimally part of the thinking given that the foundation was not interested in creating "new" nonprofit agencies.[8]

Program Design Phase

The Colorado Rural Health Center (CRHC) was selected, through a competitive bid process, to manage VRSI. At the time that CRHC was selected, several basic program elements had not been specified. These included defining what is "rural," defining who is a "volunteer," and determining how large individual grants should be, for what duration, and for what types of services.

In its proposal, CRHC offered to establish an advisory committee that would work out program details. The advisory committee consisted of 12 individuals representing organizations ranging from AARP, to the Colorado Department of Public Health and Environment, to several service providers.

In preparing to issue its first request for proposals in 1996, CRHC staff and the advisory committee fleshed out program parameters:

- "Rural" Colorado was defined to include all of the 52 counties that lie outside the state's Standard Metropolitan Statistical Areas plus all towns of less than 25,000 population (even if they were located within one of the state's 11 metropolitan counties).
- "Seniors" were defined as people 60 years of age or over.
- Although projects were required to use volunteers, what constituted being a "volunteer" was not defined. Developing an intergenerational pool of volunteers was encouraged.
- Budget requests could not exceed $25,000 per year for a 3-year period (for a total of $75,000), with smaller requests being encouraged. Proposals for new programs were given equal preference as proposals for enhancement of existing programs. All projects, however, had to be community based, meaning that they were expected to demonstrate community collaboration, support, and involvement. When multiple applicants requested funds from the same community, they were encouraged to collaborate. Those that did were funded. None of these parameters changed significantly over three subsequent rounds of awards.

Prior to the design phase, community members influenced the goals of VRSI through their responses to a statewide needs assessment effort of The

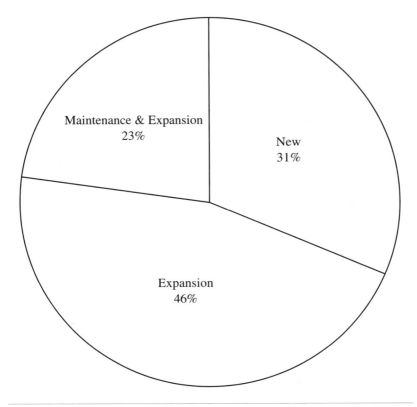

Figure 6.1   New Programs Versus Expansion Programs ($N = 35$)

Colorado Trust. Community-based organizations then submitted proposals based on criteria developed by the foundation and the managing agency in consultation with its advisory committee.

Selecting Grantees

VRSI applicants were community-based organizations, including non-profits and government agencies. Their proposals were required to include an assessment of the needs of seniors in the community along with a specification of the services to be provided. Organizations applying for grants included hospitals, city governments, schools, senior centers, and religious organizations. The relatively inclusive approach reflected a belief in the importance of building on the unique assets of individual communities and their organizations.

CRHC awarded 35 grants, of which 34 were completed. Of these grants, 11 (31%) were awarded to new programs (Figure 6.1). The number of new programs is quite high in view of the fact that VRSI was designed primarily to strengthen ongoing programs.[9] In addition, 16 grants (46%) went to

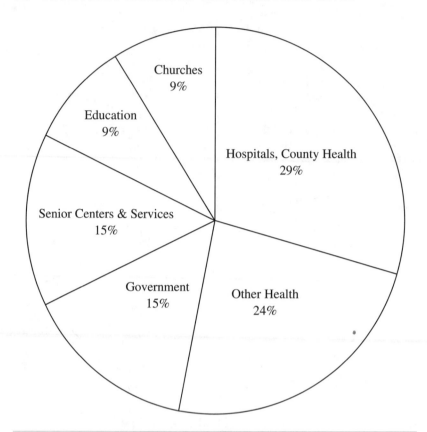

Figure 6.2   Types of Host Organizations ($N = 34$)

organizations proposing program expansions, and 8 grants (23%) either were maintaining ongoing programs or were planning to combine maintenance and expansion.

The amounts of the grants varied from $4,154 to $75,000 over a 3-year period. Although more than half of the projects requested more than $45,000, a sizable number requested under $30,000. When these grants are prorated by number of years, they were remarkably similar in size—about $15,500 per year. This is consistent with CRHC's goal of giving small grants so as to support a larger number of programs.

Although there was some variation in the types of organizations that hosted VRSI projects, 18 projects (53%) were health service organizations such as hospitals, county health departments, clinics, home health organizations, and a hospice (Figure 6.2). Two other groups included government agencies (5 projects), especially city and county governments, and senior service organizations (5 projects).

Educational institutions and churches were also host organizations. Educational organizations tended to participate as collaborating organizations initially and then often became primary hosts. Some used seniors as volunteers in the schools or as clients for their students. Churches tended to pursue short-duration grants[10] for ongoing volunteer programs for seniors such as buying a lift to carry seniors down stairs to their eating area or to lift seniors into vans to assist in meal delivery programs.

IMPLEMENTATION

Although the selection criteria were met when the managing agency awarded the funds, over time it became apparent that some of the criteria critical to creating community-based projects were being modified through the implementation process. For example, projects had to be based on a volunteer component. Although some organizations claimed (in their applications) to have a volunteer component, they actually paid volunteers for their services. Similarly, CRHC guidelines encouraged collaboration among organizations serving the same community. Some of those collaborations, however, never really developed once grants were awarded.

To examine the implementation process more closely, eight VRSI programs were selected to represent the variety of projects in the initiative and were studied in more detail (Table 6.1). These case study results are presented in the following subsections.

Start-Up Phase

Start-up issues were similar for all VRSI projects. Recruiting volunteers and marketing services were the hardest start-up issues. Project staff said that they had too little time and funding to develop needed publicity materials.[11] Ultimately, they got project information to the community through newspapers (94%), by word of mouth (77%), through health professionals (71%), and at public meetings (53%). Other major start-up issues included the challenges of managing and developing the projects. Staff were daunted by the need to develop project forms, documentation, and other management tools. These created "snafus and time glitches that have us on temporary hold," a staffer explained (Lodwick & Wallis, 1996a).

Survey findings showed that 77% of the grantees reported using word of mouth as their primary volunteer recruitment strategy. Newspaper (53%), radio (35%), and newsletters (29%) were also used by a sizable number of the projects (Lodwick & Wallis, 1996b). Many VRSI coordinators said that they had not realized the complexity and demands of managing a volunteer-based program before their projects got under way.

Table 6.1   Characteristics of Eight VRSI Case Studies

	Start-Up			Operations				Sustainability	
Case Study	Type of Host/ Program	Marketing	Service Type	Volunteers	Seniors	Niche Issues	Turf Issues	Host's Support	Resources
Meeker	Health and county/ ongoing capital improvement	Hospital referral, newspaper, word of mouth	Transportation, meal delivery	About 12 adults, ongoing	Fragile seniors with low support network	None	None	Ongoing support; subsidizes meals at $20,000/year	Ongoing from the hospital and the county; community pride and support
Wray	Health and recreation/ ongoing capital improvement	Newspaper, word of mouth, senior information display center	Warm water therapy (chemicals), senior information (display), door opening (handles)	Community service organizations	Active and fragile seniors.	None	None	Not relevant for capital improvement	Ongoing program fund-raising
Cortez	Health/new	Newspaper, referrals from hospital and health department, word of mouth, speakers	Teacher aide in elementary schools, home visits, respite, transportation, errands	Year 1: 4; Year 2: 8; Year 3: 15; healthy seniors, adults, and staff	Year 1: 7; Year 2: 23; Year 3: 25; fragile, homebound, active seniors	Who evaluates and pays seniors for the schools? What is value added for paying VRSI coordinator rather than social worker?	Program focus and volunteer use—senior center; no student volunteers— school; volunteers' use—church	Schools became program hosts; health department reduced support	School paid seniors in one program

| | Start-Up | | Operations | | | Sustainability | | | |
Case Study	Type of Host/ Program	Marketing	Service Type	Volunteers	Seniors	Niche Issues	Turf Issues	Host's Support	Resources
Haxtun	Health and school/new	Town newsletter, word of mouth, speakers	Chores, yard work, home visits, home maintenance, delivery, transportation	Year 1: 0 youth and 7 adults; Year 2:16 youth and 7 adults; Year 3: 20 youth and 23 adults	Year 1: 7; Year 2: 27; Year 3: 34; both active and fragile, homebound seniors	Most support from school, referrals, and office from host hospital	Use of volunteers and program focus of Area Agency on Aging	School in Fleming became host; hospital referral and housing host	School and church contributions; hospital referrals; grants
Fountain	Senior services/new	Word of mouth, announcements at senior center	Sitter, yard work, home maintenance, telephone visits, respite	Year 1: 67, 50/5 youth and some men; Year 2: 98 youth, seniors, and other adults	Year 1: 81; Year 2: 127	Program funds	None	Supportive but no funds	Grant writing; fund-raising
Fairplay	Senior services/ ongoing	Newspaper, newsletter, word of mouth, mail carrier, speakers, announcements	Newsletter, transportation, homemaker, CPA tax assistance, newsletter, handyman, more programs, transportation	Year 1: 57; Year 2: 80; Year 3: 80+; board members, seniors, and family members	Seniors as volunteers and clients; mostly healthy seniors (22)	New coordinators hired	Leadership challenge and overlap of volunteers; senior center	Supportive	Federal grants; collaborating organizations

(Continued)

Table 6.1 Continued

| | | Start-Up | | Operations | | | Sustainability | | |
Case Study	Type of Host/Program	Marketing	Service Type	Volunteers	Seniors	Niche Issues	Turf Issues	Host's Support	Resources
Alamosa	Senior services and education/ongoing	Word of mouth, senior center announcements	Transportation, homemaker, walking program	Year 1: 15; Year 2: 26; Year 3: 26; nurses and medical interns, students; and homemakers	Year 1: 6; Year 2: 27; Year 3: 22; active and some fragile seniors	None	Ongoing expansion	Ongoing strong support	Ongoing medical and nursing interns; grants
Fort Lupton	School/ongoing capital improvement	None	Construction of walkway	A few helped with construction and landscaping	None	None	None	Capital improvement	Not relevant

NOTE: VRSI = Volunteers for Rural Seniors Initiative.

132

Turnover in the director or coordinator position occurred in more than half of the VRSI projects (19 of 34), primarily during the start-up period. Loss of project leadership at this critical time contributed to loss of funds and slower program start-up because the replacements had not been involved in previous program design discussions.

Host Organizations

A host is an organization that takes the lead in making a grant application and in subsequently administering a program. Host organizations were critical in several ways. If a program required collaboration with other agencies, the host took the lead in bringing the collaboration together and making it work. The host often supplemented grant resources with in-kind donations, especially of staff support and space. Some hosts had existing volunteer programs to build on. All had visibility in the community that could help provide credibility for the new programs and their staff.

If a VRSI program was new, finding a place for it within the host organization could create a *niche* problem, that is, determining where it fit in the organization. When the missions of the host and of the VRSI program were consistent with each other, the host was often more willing to contribute its resources to nurture the project. Moreover, if the project director was part of the ongoing staff of the host rather than someone hired externally, fewer internal niche struggles were likely to occur. However, if the program was new to the host and outside of its core mission, the VRSI program had to rely more exclusively on funds brought in by the grant. The staff person hired to run it might have difficulty in being accepted as a member of the host organization.

Distinct from niche challenges, new programs can also face issues of *turf*, that is, defining where they fit in the larger community. Turf struggles with organizations in the broader community were less likely to occur if a VRSI grant simply expanded or maintained an ongoing program. In contrast, other community-based organizations working with volunteers or with seniors in the community would respond negatively to a new program that sought to provide volunteer-based services to seniors. Within the case study communities, initial struggles tended to center around issues of potential duplication of services and of volunteer use.

The characteristics of the host organization also affected whether or not a VRSI program had easy access to volunteers and seniors. Health-based hosts had plenty of seniors who needed services but had no volunteer group to draw on. In contrast, senior service centers often had access to seniors and experience with volunteers but faced difficulties in matching what volunteers wanted to do with the needs of seniors. Education-based organizations often had volunteers but had to develop a senior clientele base. Churches served as referral and volunteer sources while tending to serve primarily their own members.

Start-up issues such as these were especially daunting for new programs. New VRSI programs were challenged to train new personnel, discover their niche in the host organizations, develop their turf in the wider communities, develop program support and advertisement materials, recruit seniors, and recruit and train volunteers. These were huge tasks for new directors or coordinators, who typically had little experience in working with volunteers and seniors.

Operations Phase

One of the critical activities of the second year for programs was to create an appropriate fit between the capacities and interests of volunteers, on the one hand, and the needs of seniors, on the other. This struggle was apparent in two projects. In the first, a health department originally planned to build a cadre of adult volunteers to supplement a home health care program for their many homebound senior clients. However, one senior convinced the department to add a program to the VRSI grant proposal that would involve having seniors work as volunteers in the local elementary schools. When the proposal was funded, most of the program coordinator's time during the first year went into working on the school program rather than on the home care program.

By the second year of the program, seniors had been placed in four of five elementary schools. The seniors had monthly meetings, their own T-shirts, and their own identity. They supported each other both formally and informally, felt valued, and "had a purpose for getting up in the morning." Most of them saw this as a "job" with attendant responsibilities.[12]

Meanwhile, the host organization continued to have difficulties in recruiting volunteers to serve the homebound frail seniors who had been the original target clientele of its grant. Even though the VRSI program paid mileage and provided special training to volunteers, these incentives were not sufficient to develop and retain volunteers for the homebound elderly.

During the second year of the project, there were only three nonstaff volunteers in the homebound elderly program. The director of the health department and other staff became active as "volunteers." They ran errands for clients, took them to medical appointments, and provided other volunteer services. The program coordinator was kept busy trying to find volunteers to serve as many as 23 homebound seniors, and her position was increased to full-time. Efforts to recruit volunteers in churches met with little success. While program demands increased, the hosting health department became increasingly dissatisfied with the program's inability to meet "its" seniors' needs. The department was not receiving the benefits it had expected from the program.

The health department then sought to meet its clients' increasing demands by hiring an adult protection specialist who worked with homebound and other elders, the first such position in the region. With the hiring of this specialist, the volunteer coordinator's position was reduced. In terms of the overall "success" of the project, the host's director reported that having a volunteer program changed the culture of the health department to be more sensitive to senior needs than was the case prior to VRSI. The director also believed that there were insufficient volunteer resources to support the needs of the homebound elderly.

A second VRSI project had a more successful second year. During the first year, most of the nine volunteers were high school students who needed to complete a community service requirement for graduation. The primary services they provided were home chores and yard cleanup. The seven senior citizens who received services from the program during the first year explained their acceptance of the volunteer services as their way of supporting the young people's graduation requirements rather than as a way of meeting their own needs.

During the second year, the program continued to work primarily with young volunteers while gradually recruiting adult volunteers. By the end of the year, the program had about 16 volunteers, including 7 adults, providing services to 27 seniors.

In both of these examples, the programs struggled to match the abilities and interests of the volunteers with the needs of the seniors. In one VRSI program, vigorous seniors wanted to work with students but not with fragile homebound seniors. In the second case study, senior clients agreed to accept what services young volunteers could provide to help the students meet school requirements.

A clear lesson from these cases is that volunteer programs are often not implemented as designed because the capacities and interests of the volunteer pool are usually not known until recruiting begins. A second lesson is that there are challenges in trying to match the abilities of the volunteers with the types of clients to whom volunteer services are being directed. Only some of the mismatch[13] between volunteers' capacities/interests and seniors' needs can be remedied with training.

Changes in Community Support

Many VRSI programs actively sought community support as they attempted to balance the abilities and interests of volunteers with the needs of seniors. They resolved turf issues and developed community outreach. Directors or coordinators were often key to the outreach, increasing their speaking engagements or working with other community-based groups to inform the community of services and the need for volunteers. In so doing, they often created a more general increased awareness of and support for seniors in the community.

In one case, a coordinator increased her presentations to community social groups, churches, and other organizations. One church responded by raising funds to help support the program. Another church developed a monthly program for seniors. As the program expanded, turf issues emerged when another senior agency became concerned that the VRSI program would compete for local volunteers. The VRSI coordinator then applied her efforts to pursuing additional grants rather than recruiting additional senior volunteers. She wrote and received a Robert Wood Johnson grant to hire a local assistant in another town. She also helped a local congregation to apply for and receive a handicapped accessibility grant. Through these efforts, she helped the community to give higher priority to senior issues.

In another VRSI community, turf issues developed between a senior center and the VRSI program over leadership issues. The two programs had collaborated in purchasing and refurbishing a building for the senior center. When the senior center's president left for the winter, as is common in that region, the seniors turned to the VRSI coordinator for leadership. This created bitterness among some seniors who believed that the VRSI coordinator was trying to take over the senior center, creating only one senior-serving organization. This conflict was eventually resolved through negotiations.

Other community organizations became more involved with senior issues as VRSI program seniors asked service clubs, churches, and other organizations to help provide volunteer services. An elementary school began having monthly breakfasts for seniors who helped in the school's reading program. As VRSI communities focused on the contributions of seniors, a more general trend observed was that of community-based organizations increasing their collaborations with the seniors in planning services for the community as a whole.

Sustainability Phase

The main challenge of the third and final year of the grant was to find resources to continue providing services to seniors. Four strategies used by VRSI programs were that (a) the host organization accepted responsibility for sustaining the program, (b) another organization or group of organizations agreed to sustain the services, (c) the services of the program were redistributed among different organizations, and (d) the services and program were discontinued.

In one VRSI community, a host organization used the VRSI grant to strengthen its infrastructure and to generate more funds to sustain and increase the program. The director used VRSI funds to professionalize the bookkeeping and volunteer tracking systems, to hire new site coordinators, and to professionalize their communication and planning. He also enhanced communication with the seniors in the county and developed a stronger senior self-governance system. In this site, collaboration was also strengthened with major institutions in the county—education, churches, and county commissioners. The strengthened program increased its resources with a "wellness grant" and with federal grants because of its work on volunteer tracking and organizing. When assessing VRSI's impact, the director said,

> We have established a critical mass of seniors and others involved in the program. We have become more volunteer focused and less director led. People are also more aware of senior needs.[14]

Given these positive developments, this host organization will sustain the volunteer program even after VRSI funds are no longer available.

In another grantee community, a city government agreed to fund a senior outreach position at the end of the VRSI grant period. By highlighting the demand for senior services, the VRSI program increased the city government's response to those needs. The host organization was willing to contribute programmatic infrastructure for the volunteer program, while the city provided funds to maintain the outreach position. In this instance, therefore, another organization agreed to sustain the services.

In the final example, the VRSI grant was used to fund two very different programs that were administered by a single host organization: (a) VRSI senior teaching aides and (b) homebound senior visitors. At the end of the grant, the teacher aides were sustained by a school district, and the homebound seniors program was dissolved. Therefore, some of the services were discontinued, while the others were sustained.

Being able to sustain efforts was most critical for new organizations. Ongoing community organizations, in contrast, simply expanded or decreased programmatic functions based on funding or on how they were able to sustain the services. In the more successful organizations, these sustainability efforts were accompanied by increases in community awareness and support for seniors.

Initiative Outcomes and Impacts

How well did VRSI succeed in meeting its objectives? The two basic types of evaluations that help to answer this question are outcome and impact evaluations.

OUTCOMES

Outcomes are the consequences resulting directly and immediately from program activities. If a program activity is recruitment, an outcome measure is

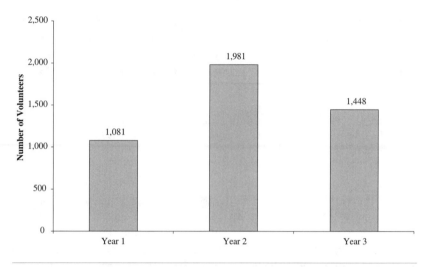

Figure 6.3   Volunteers Over 3 Years

NOTE: Figure includes only data from organizations for which data were available for all 3 years.

the number of volunteers actually recruited. Similarly, if an activity is designed to provide services to seniors, outcome measures include the range of services provided to a specific number of seniors. Principal areas where outcomes are of interest include volunteers, services, and clients.

Volunteers

Across VRSI, 29 reporting programs were supported by the efforts of more than 2,000 volunteers. Over the 3 years of the VRSI projects, volunteers provided a total monthly average of 11,682 hours of service.

The number of volunteers varied across phases of program development. For the purpose of seeing the changes across time, only those organizations providing information for all 3 years were included in the analysis. During the first year, when many programs were focused largely on start-up activities, these programs had a total of 1,081 volunteers providing a monthly average of 3,882 hours of service (Figures 6.3 and 6.4). By the second year of the programs, the success of volunteer recruitment and retention efforts led these programs to have a total of 1,981 volunteers, an increase of 83% over the first year. That year, volunteers provided a total monthly average of 13,962 hours of service. By the final year of the program, staff attention focused on challenges of sustainability, and the number of volunteers declined by 34% to 1,448 from the previous-year high. However, there were still 34% more volunteers during the final year of these programs than during the first year, providing 9,518 monthly hours of service.

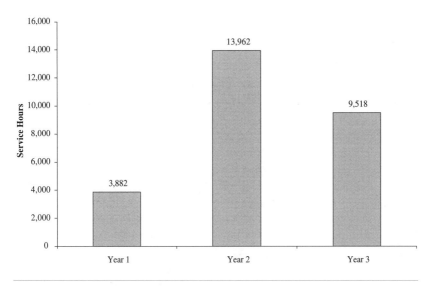

Figure 6.4   Average Monthly Service Hours Over 3 Years

NOTE: Figure includes only data from organizations for which data were available for all 3 years.

Across all VRSI sites, the majority (58%) of volunteers were seniors, 30% were working-age adults, and the rest were under 21 years of age. Over the 3 years, the number of senior volunteers decreased by 12%, the percentage of working-age adults remained steady, and the number of volunteers under 21 years of age increased by 56%.

Services and Clients

VRSI programs offered 10 different kinds of services (Figure 6.5). Some sites offered only one service, but most offered several. Meal delivery and preparation accounted for 35% of all volunteer time. Personal visits (13%), transportation (9%), and home chores and maintenance (8%) ranked second, third, and fourth, respectively. A mixture of "other" services comprised 12% of all volunteer hours. In addition, 14% of the service hours were dedicated to program management, fund-raising, and advertising.

As mentioned previously, volunteer hours varied over the 3 years. In addition, they varied by service. Transportation, education and information, home chores, and maintenance increased continuously over VRSI. On the other hand, meal delivery and preparation and personal visits declined during the third year. Presumably, service areas that continued to grow over the initiative

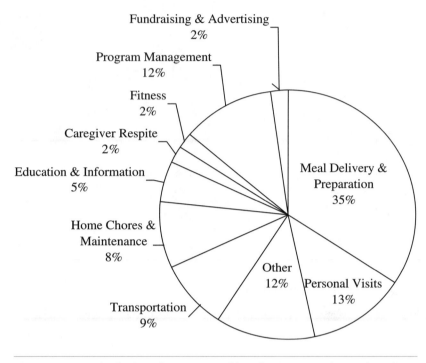

Figure 6.5   Distribution of Average Monthly Volunteer Hours (11,682 hours)

were meeting needs that had not been fully met. Others, such as meal delivery, have inherent constraints such as regular travel time requirements.

Fully 85% of the VRSI program clients were seniors, whereas 15% were not (Figure 6.6). About equal percentages of seniors were young (ages 60–74 years) and old (age 75 years or over) (43% and 42%, respectively).

Did VRSI Funds Make a Difference?

As part of the evaluation, telephone interviews were conducted with staff from eight organizations that had applied for VRSI funding but had not won grants. The principal objective of the interviews was to determine whether these programs had proceeded in the absence of grant funding. Responses suggest that applicants seeking funds to expand or enhance ongoing programs continued to conduct those programs, although often without any of the proposed changes. In contrast, those organizations that were proposing to start new programs did not follow through on those plans in the absence of grants.

To test whether VRSI made a difference, the eight senior organizations that were unsuccessful in applying for VRSI funds were compared with eight

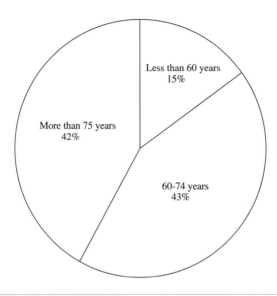

Figure 6.6   VRSI Client Ages (3,729 clients)

matched VRSI grantees. Five of the eight VRSI organizations were able to increase their communities' resources to meet senior needs, whereas only two nonawarded organizations were also able to do so during the same period. In the case of programs receiving funds to start new programs, the impact of VRSI grants is less ambiguous. Organizations that did not receive grants did not develop programs, whereas those that received grants did.

IMPACTS

The ultimate impacts that The Colorado Trust sought in establishing VRSI was to use volunteers to help seniors successfully stay in their homes longer than they would otherwise be able to do. To achieve this outcome, not only would community-based organizations have to generate a sufficient number of volunteers, but those volunteers would have to be able to deliver the right kinds of services on a timely and sustained basis. It is difficult to determine whether this type of impact occurred because measuring it would require a long-term perspective necessitating evaluation well after the end of the initiative. Nevertheless, some findings are evident, even in the near term.

The reasons why seniors move out of their homes include the death of their spouses, major changes in friends or neighborhoods, accidents (e.g., a broken hip), disrepair of their homes that reduces habitability, and increased and progressive frailness (Norris-Baker & Scheidt, 1994; Rowles, 1983). The

Table 6.2   Changes in Social Contacts of VRSI ($n = 12$) and Comparison
($n = 13$) Seniors

	VRSI Seniors	Comparison Seniors
Friends network		
Less	4	1
Same	5	7
More	3	4
Family network		
Less	1	2
Same	6	4
More	4	5

NOTE: VRSI = Volunteers for Rural Seniors Initiative.

services that VRSI volunteers could provide were (for the most part) modest but were not insignificant in assisting seniors in some of these situations.

Delivering meals, while simultaneously providing a brief respite of companionship, was greatly appreciated and satisfied a clear and significant need. But programs also delivered meals to seniors who found it a convenience rather than a necessity. The work of volunteers in providing modest home maintenance, such as installing bathroom grab bars and replacing light bulbs, was in some cases essential to keeping the seniors' homes safe and habitable. But service in tidying up lawns had a more modest effect, if any, on maintaining people in their homes, although it improved the quality of life for the seniors.[15]

For the most part, the services provided could help seniors who were suffering episodic disabilities such as recovering from operations. Volunteers could also attend to house repair problems that were minor but nevertheless annoying and even hazardous to the occupants. Personal visits, sometimes accompanied with delivery of meals, provided support to people suffering from the loss of their spouses or, more generally, from the loss of companionship. In general, however, these services were far too modest to provide the support required by people with progressive and significant frailness.

Impacts on Seniors

In trying to determine the impacts of VRSI programs, changes in health, social relations, and quality of life factors of seniors who received VRSI services were compared with those of seniors who did not receive these services. Two sets of in-depth interviews were conducted approximately 1 year apart with clients and paired nonclients in two communities (Table 6.2).

Table 6.3   Changes in Health and Other Indicators of VRSI ($n = 20$) and Comparison ($n = 19$) Seniors

	VRSI Seniors	Comparison Seniors
Health		
Worse	11	10
Same	8	8
Better	1	1
Number of medicines		
More	6	2
Same	10	9
Less	4	8
Activities of daily living		
Worse	5	4
Same	11	9
Better	4	6
Health care provider visits		
More	10	5
Same	7	8
Less	3	6
Housing*		
Worse	7	1
Same	13	14
Better	0	4
Transportation		
Worse	9	4
Same	11	15
Better	0	0

NOTE: VRSI = Volunteers for Rural Seniors Initiative. By the second panel, 1 VRSI senior had died. Of the comparison seniors, 2 moved, 1 died, and 4 were not known.
*Significant difference between VRSI and comparison seniors at the .05 level.

Overall, both groups of seniors reported that their health deteriorated during the interval between interviews. Contacts with family members increased for both groups during that period. VRSI clients reported seeing friends and neighbors less than they did the previous year, whereas nonclients reported more frequent contacts with neighbors (Table 6.3).

The only statistically significant difference between the two groups during the 1-year time period was further deterioration of their homes, with VRSI clients reporting more deterioration in their housing. Clients also mentioned deterioration of transportation (e.g., giving up driving or significantly limiting it) more frequently than did nonclients. Health indicators remained similar for both groups.

Most senior clients appreciated the services that they received through the VRSI program, although many did not understand the connection between the volunteers and the local VRSI office. When seniors received services from young volunteers, they found the experience rewarding, in part because they believed that they could offer some mentoring in return or at least provide some refreshments. They also became better acquainted with young people in their communities and enjoyed their "fresh viewpoints." Senior clients who became paid volunteers as teacher aides enjoyed the experience and found that it helped to improve their self-esteem.

Program coordinators were also interviewed and questioned about ways in which they believed the lives of seniors had been affected by VRSI services. Sometimes programs indirectly helped to maintain seniors at home. Some of the ways mentioned by program staff included helping a client to obtain hearing aids so that she felt safe driving to the grocery store, providing transportation to a hospital to help keep two senior friends together until one died, and constructing a wheelchair ramp so that a caregiver could take a senior outside.

Impacts on Volunteers

Focus groups and interviews were conducted with volunteers in the same communities where clients were interviewed. Volunteers uniformly described their experiences in working with seniors as rewarding. Many senior men shared that they had not done volunteer work before getting involved in the VRSI program. Women, in contrast, often had prior volunteering experience.[16]

Youth participating in VRSI programs often had little or no prior volunteering experience. These youth tended to be brought into volunteering as the result of a graduation requirement. Nevertheless, many youth viewed the opportunity of working with seniors as a way of bridging a generation gap. Seniors similarly enjoyed the opportunity to meet youth.

In interviews with working adults and with VRSI program staff, an interesting pattern was identified. They suggested that most working adults are able to give some volunteer time but that it has become more limited as both husbands and wives find it necessary to be employed. Consequently, when these people volunteer, they prefer not to make long-term or extensive commitments. Helping to winterize homes over a weekend or giving 20 hours of community service as a graduation requirement works within the schedules of the new volunteers.[17] In contrast, the idea of committing even 1 hour per week to meal delivery on an ongoing basis is far more difficult to make.

The experience of VRSI programs confirms that there is a pool of untapped volunteers available in rural communities. At the same time, these results suggest that volunteering for many is more of an episodic commitment than a long-term one. Consequently, ongoing recruitment of this community resource is essential for sustaining volunteer involvement.

Impacts on Communities and Organizations

At the community level, a desired impact of VRSI would be heightened awareness of the needs of seniors. There is largely anecdotal evidence at this point of modest change along this dimension in participating VRSI communities. Program coordinators repeated stories suggesting a relative insensitivity to the needs of seniors in rural communities. They maintained that there was now greater awareness of those needs. Some cited examples of this such as unexpected groups contributing to their programs, health fairs that included an emphasis on senior issues, funding made available for staff positions, and greater response to the transportation needs of seniors.

The evidence of organizational-level impacts is more apparent. Many of the community-based organizations that applied for VRSI grants already had missions focusing on serving the needs of seniors, but some did not. A hospital or health district nominally serves all citizens of a community, with no particular emphasis on seniors. In addition, after grants were awarded, several programs managed to find additional collaborators that had no previous mission focus on seniors (e.g., schools).

From a short-term perspective, it is difficult to determine whether participating organizations will sustain their new or heightened commitment to serving seniors. Grant funds provide an artificial stimulus to participation that may disappear as funding expires. But in a very few cases, VRSI personnel have been picked up and new programs have been incorporated within organizations' full range of activities.

Thus, there are some indications that the VRSI grants did stimulate community-based organizations to generate additional community resources to address a previously obscured community need. Some communities embraced and sustained the efforts, whereas in others the programs disappeared at the end of the grant period.

Lessons Learned

Overall, this evaluation found that VRSI met its objectives. It stimulated the expansion and development of services to rural seniors through the use of volunteers. Grantees demonstrated that there is an untapped reserve of volunteers who can be engaged for this purpose. In addition, the kinds of services provided succeeded in improving the quality of life of those served. Although these volunteer services were modest and incapable of compensating for major episodes (e.g., a broken hip, significant home maintenance problems) that would force seniors out of their independent living arrangements, VRSI was not intended to address major kinds of crises.

Some of the more specific lessons learned are listed in what follows in two areas: (a) program outcomes and impacts and (b) program design and implementation.

PROGRAM OUTCOMES AND IMPACTS

Funding helps to stimulate community awareness of the needs of seniors. There is a widening gap between the needs of seniors and the capacity of rural communities to satisfy those needs. Funding community-based organizations helps to raise community awareness of those needs and motivates the generation of resources to address them.

New programs can tap unused reserves of volunteers. The success of VRSI programs in finding volunteers suggests that there is an untapped reserve of such labor in rural communities. Indeed, many volunteers were new to the practice of giving their time in this form of service rather than solely through helping behavior. It seems especially important to stimulate an ethic of volunteering among teenagers, thereby building a bridge across generations.

New programs may raise turf protection responses by existing volunteer-based programs. New volunteer programs introduced in a community are likely to provoke a *turf* protection response from other volunteer agencies that may become concerned about competition. Independent of the use of volunteers, other senior-serving providers might feel that their territory is being encroached on. Recognizing these possibilities, program personnel and senior administrators or board members with the host organization should explain the objectives of a new program to allay concerns, preferably before the program formally begins.

The use of volunteers makes programs more truly community based. Using younger seniors to design and implement programs to serve both younger and older seniors makes the programs truly community based. It also increases community awareness of the needs of seniors. Similarly, using an intergenerational mix of volunteers has a positive effect on the quality of life for both the volunteers and the recipients.

Volunteer skills and senior needs are often mismatched. Matching the skills and interests of volunteers with the needs of seniors has proven to be difficult. This was especially evident in VRSI programs designed to provide visits to frail seniors or to offer respite care. Carefully matching the skills and interests of volunteers with clients' needs, as well as training, may help to improve the fit. However, most programs focused on recruiting as many volunteers as they could and ended up redefining the services they provided to clients based on what their volunteers could do.

Sustained effort is necessary to establish and maintain formal volunteer-based programs. Small grants can be effective in stimulating volunteer-based programs to work with a greater number of seniors in rural areas. At the same time, the changing nature of volunteering requires ongoing efforts at recruitment and retention. These efforts may be aided by having clear program identity and staffing rather than having services that are less clearly identifiable among a panoply of other offerings by a host organization.

PROGRAM DESIGN AND IMPLEMENTATION

Funding new programs most clearly demonstrates program impacts. VRSI funds had their clearest and least ambiguous outcomes and impacts when applied to new programs rather than to supporting existing programs. Yet existing programs were found to have the greatest probability of being sustained. This presents a real trade-off, and funders need to be clear regarding their objective, whether it is stimulating new programs or sustaining established ones.

Organizational capacity should be a key criterion in selecting grantees. In selecting grant recipients, it is important to consider organizational capacity as well as the alignment of organizational mission with the goals of the grant program. Organizations in which the alignment between the general organizational goals and the specific VRSI program needs were weak encountered significant *niche* challenges, that is, questions about where they fit in and whether they were necessary. At the same time, it is important to award grants to organizations that have strong credibility in their communities, even if they have no history of providing services to seniors.

Provide program staff with many opportunities to network with one another. The staffs of newly established programs, who are likely to be new to their organizations as well, benefit from opportunities to network with their counterparts in similar programs elsewhere. Networking helps to provide staff with resources to think through new challenges such as how to advertise a program. Networking can similarly help to ensure program sustainability.

It is important to be clear about what is meant by a volunteer-based program. Some programs maintained that it was appropriate to pay volunteers if they had limited means. This practice raised the question as to whether all grantees understood what it means to be a "volunteer" and whether the culture of helping in rural areas might be changing as the result of demographic changes.

Seniors who are newcomers to rural communities seem to find it easier to volunteer and receive the services of volunteers, whereas old-timers remain more independent and suspicious of formalized volunteering.

VRSI demonstrated how stimulating the participation of appropriate community-based organizations can generate capacity to identify and address the needs of an underserved segment of the community. Sustaining such programs after funding ends, however, was found to be a difficult challenge. To be sustained, new programs in particular will need to have created a clear identity and value that is supported by their communities. Only then will a health promotion effort such as this be fully community based.

Notes

1. Interviews conducted during central site visits in 1997 and 1998.
2. Interviews conducted in northeast area in 1997 and 1998.
3. Interviews conducted in northeast area in 1997 and 1998.
4. VRSI was designed to stimulate development of complementary volunteer assistance to medical and other professional services.
5. The pattern of disengagement was reported in Rowles (1983).
6. Interviews conducted during central site visits in 1997 and 1998.
7. Freedman (1997) describes how senior volunteers are critical as "community keepers." They are especially open to working with youth.
8. Interview with program officer on December 6, 1999.
9. This created quite a challenge for CRHC to learn how to best support the new programs.
10. Of the three grants, only one was for 2 years and the other two were for 1 year.
11. In a study of 100 volunteer programs offering ongoing handyman repair services, fix-up or seasonal programs, or intergenerational programs, Osterkamp and Chapin (1995) find this to be a recurring concern.
12. Cnaan and Cwikel (1992) examine the types of services that seniors preferred to contribute as volunteers and find that they preferred "meaningful assignments that involved interpersonal communication" (p. 139). Freedman (1997) reports that "helping the younger generation is the greatest preference seniors have for volunteer work" (p. 249).
13. Cnaan and Cwikel (1992) warn about the potential incompatibility between the interests of senior volunteers and agency needs.
14. Interview with a program coordinator in 1998.
15. This conclusion was also reached by Osterkamp and Chapin (1995).
16. This is consistent with Cnaan and Cwikel (1992) but inconsistent with Wilson and Musick (1997).
17. Osterkamp and Chapin (1995) propose ways of combining the orientations of the volunteers to increase community awareness and involvement with seniors.

References

Amato, P. (1993). Urban rural differences in helping friends and family members. *Social Psychology Quarterly, 56,* 249–262.

Cnaan, R. A., & Cwikel, J. G. (1992). Elderly volunteers: Assessing their potential as an untapped resource. *Journal of Aging and Social Policy, 4*(1/2), 25–147.

Freedman, M. (1997). Toward civic renewal: How senior citizens could save civil society. *Journal of Gerontological Social Work, 28,* 243–263.

Lodwick, D. G., & Wallis, A. (1996a). *Quarterly Report–3: Volunteers for Rural Seniors Initiative.* Denver: The Colorado Trust.

Lodwick, D. G., & Wallis, A. (1996b). *Quarterly Report–4: Volunteers for Rural Seniors Initiative.* Denver: The Colorado Trust.

Minkler, M. (1997). *Community organizing and community building for health.* New Brunswick, NJ: Rutgers University Press.

Norris-Baker, C., & Scheidt, R. J. (1994). From "our town" to "ghost town"? The changing context of home for rural elders. *International Journal of Aging and Human Development, 38,* 181–202.

Osterkamp, L. B., & Chapin, R. (1995). Community-based volunteer home-repair and home-maintenance programs for elders: An effective service paradigm? *Journal of Gerontological Social Work, 24*(1/2), 55–75.

Rowles, G. (1983). Between worlds: A relocation dilemma for the Appalachian elderly. *International Journal of Aging and Human Development, 17,* 301–331.

Wilson, J., & Musick, M. (1997). Who cares? Towards an integrated theory of volunteer work. *American Sociological Review, 62,* 694–713.

7

The Colorado School Health Education Initiative

Promoting School Health Education Through Capacity Building

Deborah S. Main

Douglas H. Fernald

Kathryn A. Judge Nearing

Donna K. Duffy

Jill A. Elnicki

The majority of illnesses, deaths, and social problems among young people are caused by a relatively few preventable health behaviors. According to the Centers for Disease Control and Prevention (CDC, 2000), the leading causes of morbidity and mortality among youth ages 10 to 24 years in the United States are as follows:

- Unintentional injuries
- Tobacco use

- Alcohol or other drug use
- Sexual behaviors that lead to unintentional pregnancy and sexually transmitted diseases
- Dietary behaviors
- Physical activity

Results of national surveys of children and adolescents indicate that youth engage in these health risk behaviors at alarming rates, with the onset for many of these behaviors beginning at progressively earlier ages. Youth are clearly an important target group for comprehensive health education that exposes them to prevention messages before they contemplate, or actually engage in, high-risk behaviors such as those identified by the 1997 Youth Risk Behavior Survey (CDC, 1998).

In the United States, millions of youth ages 5 to 17 years attend elementary and secondary schools for approximately 6 hours a day, 180 days a year. With dropout rates nearly nonexistent until high school, schools are an important vehicle for addressing the health and social problems in our nation's youth. According to the Carnegie Council on Adolescent Development, "Schools could do more than perhaps any other single institution in society to help young people, and the adults they will become, to live healthier, longer, more satisfying, and more productive lives" (quoted in CDC, 2001, p. 1).

The Healthy People 2000 national health objectives highlight the important role of schools and school health education in promoting the health of youth (National Center for Health Statistics, 1999). Specifically, one school health objective is aimed at "increas[ing] to at least 75% the proportion of the Nation's elementary and secondary schools that provide planned and sequential kindergarten–12th grade comprehensive school health education" (p. 99). Eight other objectives encourage schools to deliver categorical health education content related to nutrition, tobacco, alcohol and other drugs, sexuality, conflict resolution skills, injury prevention, HIV, and sexually transmitted diseases. The Institute of Medicine at the National Academy of Sciences also reiterates the importance of school health education, defining what a comprehensive K–12 program would look like:

A comprehensive school health program is an integrated set of planned, sequential, school-affiliated strategies, activities, and services designed to promote the optimal physical, emotional, social, and educational development of students. The program involves and is supportive of families and is determined by the local community based on community needs, resources, standards, and requirements. It is coordinated by a multidisciplinary team and [is] accountable to the community for program quality and effectiveness. (quoted in Allensworth, Lawson, Nicholson, & Wyche, 1997, p. 60)

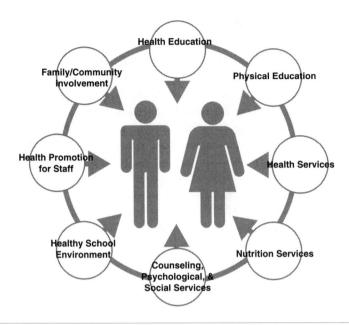

Figure 7.1   The Eight Components of a Comprehensive School Health
Program

SOURCE: *Coordinated School Health Programs: The CDC Eight Component Model of School
Health Programs.* Retrieved May 4, 2000, from www.cdc.gov/nccdphp/dash/cshpdef.htm

Figure 7.1 illustrates the eight-component model for coordinated school
health programs as defined by CDC.

In Colorado, as in many other states, school districts have struggled to put
in place comprehensive health programs as described by the Institute of
Medicine. Existing school health education programs tend to be piecemeal and
uncoordinated, are often not theoretically grounded or research based, and are
commonly given little time and attention in an increasingly stretched school
curriculum (Allensworth et al., 1997; Joint Committee on National Health
Education Standards, 1995). During a time when local school districts see
rising rates of violence, tobacco use, injury, teen pregnancy, and other risk
behaviors among youth, the role of comprehensive school health education in
enhancing the health and well-being of Colorado children has become even
more important.

Initiative Description

In 1994, in response to the scarcity of districtwide comprehensive school health education programs in the state, The Colorado Trust created a 5-year, $6.5 million initiative, the Colorado School Health Education Initiative (CSHEI). The Rocky Mountain Center for Health Promotion and Education (RMC), which served as the managing agency for the initiative, is a nonprofit organization with a 25-year history of providing staff development to school health educators across the country on research-based health education curricula. RMC has conducted curricular and assessment training for more than 20,000 people nationally and has trained teachers from more than 75% of Colorado's school districts. The RMC staff were responsible for developing the CSHEI approach to supporting school districts, disbursing grant funds to the selected districts, and providing technical assistance both to CSHEI sites and to non-CSHEI districts across Colorado.

The goals of CSHEI were as follows:

- *Develop the capacity* of local school districts to create, enhance, and/or sustain effective school health programs.
- *Increase the effectiveness* of existing school health programs in Colorado.

Although these goals provided the overarching benchmarks of program success, progress toward accomplishing these goals was to be measured through a set of more concrete objectives that could be affected and tracked during the 5 years of the CSHEI. Specifically, it was determined a priori that if the initiative were successful, schools would do the following:

- Implement effective curricula.
- Eliminate ineffective curricula.
- Teach health education at more grade levels.
- Teach health education with greater completeness and fidelity.
- Introduce other health-related programs.
- Have better trained health educators.

Two additional indicators of program success involved increasing local support for health education and reaching greater local consensus on health education programs. Both the CSHEI goals and proximal indicators were clearly defined as part of the program expectations and were integrated into its design and implementation.

CSHEI was designed to facilitate a thoughtful, planned, and inclusive approach to implementing comprehensive school health education programs. Although these programs were tailored to local needs and values, several key components were expected to be implemented in each site, including a funded health education coordinator (HEC), a health education advisory committee (HEAC), a comprehensive K–12 health education curriculum, teacher training and other professional development opportunities, and budgetary support.

The conceptual or "logic" model for CSHEI was quite simple. Namely, teachers will implement the chosen curriculum, and students will receive high-quality school health education, if each district has the following:

- A dedicated HEC to advocate for health education and support teachers
- An HEAC with improved processes for decision making and curriculum selection
- A comprehensive, research-based health education program
- Well-trained teachers to implement the health education curriculum

HEALTH EDUCATION COORDINATOR

Because local champions can be effective in mobilizing and sustaining local support for health programs (Allensworth et al., 1997; Marx, Wooley, & Northrop, 1998; Resnicow & Allensworth, 1996), CSHEI funded a health education coordinator in each site. This person was expected to increase community awareness and stakeholder participation, to facilitate curricular decision making, to link health education programs to the other components of a coordinated school health program, and to serve as a local advocate for comprehensive health education.

Each district created its own job description for the coordinator position and made the local hiring decisions. Most often, the coordinator had held a previous position in the district as a teacher, a school nurse, or an administrator. In addition to facilitating and supporting the work of the HEAC, local coordinators were expected to play key roles in the implementation of the adopted health education curriculum. The job descriptions for the HECs also called for them to organize teacher training, provide resources to teachers to supplement curricular materials, and support the regular classroom/health education teachers in implementing the adopted health education curriculum.

HEALTH EDUCATION ADVISORY COMMITTEE

A key premise of community-based health promotion is that the larger community (not just the schools) must have a voice in decision making if comprehensive school health education programs are to be implemented and sustained successfully (Allensworth et al., 1997; Bracht, 1990; Marx et al., 1998). Furthermore, staff and administrators who are asked to implement and sustain these programs must be involved in joint decision making and collaborative problem solving. Participation and commitment from a variety of stakeholders help to tailor processes and programs to address the complexities and needs specific to each site. In addition, all communities, whether rural or urban, are concerned about using school and community resources effectively and efficiently, raising the need to bring representatives of different service agencies together to avoid overlap and to ensure the coherence of services provided.

Health education advisory committees were organized to serve this role in CSHEI and were typically composed of parents, students, clergy, health and business professionals, district- and school-level administrators, teachers, and school nurses. These members were charged with setting decision-making rules and group norms, establishing the criteria for curricula selection, and determining which curricula to recommend to the school boards and other district-specific administrative committees. HEAC members also worked to develop or revise district health education standards, set goals and priorities for a coordinated school health program in the district, and advocate for health education among other community constituencies.

COMPREHENSIVE HEALTH EDUCATION CURRICULA

The HECs and the HEACs devoted the majority of their time to the processes of selecting among possible curricula, adopting the selected curriculum (i.e., gaining official approval on the part of the school district), and implementing the adopted curriculum. The RMC staff encouraged HEACs to consider curricula that are research based, theoretically driven, factually accurate, developmentally appropriate, interactive, skills based, and of sufficient duration to promote positive behavior change. Furthermore, the curricula selected should reflect local needs and values, be implemented at elementary and secondary school levels, and reinforce and build on the content taught at the previous grade level. These characteristics have been shown to be essential elements within those health education curricula that actually improve students' health-related behaviors (Dusenbury & Falco, 1995; Dusenbury & Lake, 1996; Kirby, 1997). At the same time, providing a more public forum for making curricular decisions, "as opposed to leaving such decisions to individual teachers and schools, helps ensure that curricula address essential skills and do not have redundancies or gaps [across grade levels or between schools within a district]" (Lohrmann & Wooley, 1998, p. 46). In other words, broader community-level involvement in curricular selection produces a stronger overall school health education program. To make curricular decisions within CSHEI, committees established decision-making norms and articulated the criteria by which they would evaluate different curricula.

TEACHER TRAINING AND OTHER
PROFESSIONAL DEVELOPMENT OPPORTUNITIES

Research has shown that the preparation of many teachers who provide health instruction is poor (particularly at the elementary school level) and that the use of a new health curriculum requires quality professional development (Collins et al., 1995; Joyce & Showers, 1995). Providing teacher training in adopted curricula helps to increase self-efficacy and teacher implementation. To these ends, RMC provided staff training in officially adopted curricula. Certified RMC trainers, most of whom are classroom teachers, conducted each training event, usually on-site and at no cost for the duration of sites' enrollment in CSHEI. In each district, the majority of elementary school teachers and secondary school health teachers received training at least once.

DIRECT BUDGETARY SUPPORT

CSHEI provided each site with budgetary support for the HEC position, supplemented with a small operating fund. During the first year of a site's enrollment, CSHEI funded 100% of the salary and benefits of the HEC. During subsequent years, CSHEI funding for the position decreased by 25% each year, with the CSHEI-funded districts agreeing to contribute increasing percentages of salary support to keep the coordinator position funded at its original level for the duration of the initiative (3 to 5 years, depending on when the site was enrolled). Enrolled sites received an additional annual operating budget ranging from $3,000 to $12,000, depending on the number and size of districts comprising each site. These dollars supported activities such as staff wellness, health fairs, and youth development activities. Coordinators also used these funds to cover travel expenses, attend conferences not hosted by RMC, purchase computers or office supplies, and supply food and incentives for HEAC meetings. The operating funds could not be used to support a coordinator's salary or to pay for substitute teachers when the regular classroom teachers attended trainings. (To participate in CSHEI, districts agreed to cover these costs.) The managing agency also did not fund districts to purchase selected curricula or to arrange for training. Rather, the initiative purchased these materials for each CSHEI site and sponsored training opportunities, both of which provided large financial incentives for districts that participated in the initiative.

Experience shows that for comprehensive school health programs to be adopted and sustained, they must become an integral part of what school officials think is important for children. Schools and communities, as well as state-level policymakers, must adopt a philosophy similar to that articulated by Marx et al. (1998):

> Schools can do more than perhaps any other single institution to improve the well being and competence of children and youth. Only when schools view coordinated school health programs as essential as history, social studies, or language arts will they maximize academic achievement and positive health outcomes among the children and youth they serve. (p. 298)

Within the context of CSHEI, participating schools and communities demonstrated some support for this perspective by underwriting the work of HECs, HEACs, and classroom teachers in the following:

- Reviewing and selecting health education curricula for adoption by school boards
- Providing and receiving training in these newly adopted programs
- Implementing the adopted curriculum in the classroom

ONGOING, TAILORED TECHNICAL ASSISTANCE AND SUPPORT

Because the processes of adopting, implementing, and maintaining comprehensive health education curricula varied across selected CSHEI sites, the managing agency tailored its technical assistance to meet specific district needs and the unique leadership styles of the HECs. RMC also recognized the importance of offering assistance to individuals within schools, districts, communities, and the Colorado Department of Education and Health (Chavis & Florin, 1990). Although a majority of the RMC contacts with enrolled sites took place by phone, RMC staff also traveled to CSHEI sites on an ongoing basis, providing in-person technical assistance at key points in CSHEI processes (e.g., to assist committees in establishing criteria for selecting curricula, to present different curricular options, to develop action plans for sustaining CSHEI efforts).

From the beginning, RMC dedicated some of its technical assistance energies to creating a strong network of CSHEI HECs. RMC brought HECs together at least eight times annually. Many of the coordinator meetings included workshops and skills-building sessions that focused on topics such as facilitation, preventing and managing controversy, evaluation, grant writing, leadership, social marketing, and advocacy. As the national school reform movement gained speed, RMC offered staff development training and technical assistance to districts on the use of health education standards and student performance assessment. Similarly, as the trend toward coordinated school health programs became defined, RMC began providing technical assistance and resources to help some districts explicitly link their health education programs to other components of a coordinated school health program.

Selection of Districts

To enhance the adoption, implementation, and sustainability of comprehensive health education programs, the sites selected to participate in CSHEI were those that demonstrated both high material/socioeconomic need and readiness (as described in a later section). These sites were deemed likely to receive the maximum benefits from initiative funding (Prochaska & DiClemente, 1984).

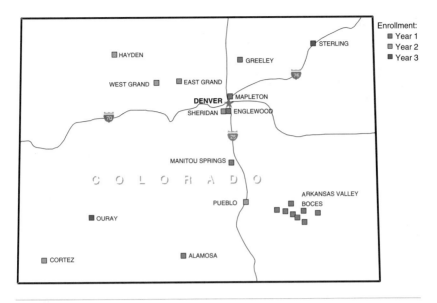

Figure 7.2   Map of CSHEI-Enrolled School Districts

Following the review of submitted "applications,"[1] letters of commitment, and site visits, as well as taking into account geographic location, RMC selected 12 sites (comprising 21 districts) to participate in CSHEI. Of these, 10 sites were single districts, 1 site consisted of a cluster of 3 districts, and 1 site consisted of an 8-district board of cooperative educational services. The largest number of sites joined the initiative during the first 2 years (6 and 4 sites in the first and second years, respectively), allowing the majority of sites to benefit maximally from the 5-year span of the initiative. The map in Figure 7.2 displays the location of districts funded by CSHEI.

Although one third (7 of 21) of selected sites/districts initially lacked an HEC, most enrolled districts rated high on many other components of infrastructure at the time they applied to participate in CSHEI. Some of these components included having an existing HEC and an active HEAC, the existence of policies supporting health education, structures in place for dealing with controversy, a history of school board support, community support for health education, and surveys conducted to collect health information.

Together, CSHEI-enrolled districts accounted for approximately 10% of the schools in Colorado and approximately 9% of students and teachers. As shown in Tables 7.1 and 7.2, per-pupil spending in CSHEI districts was typically lower than the state average, although two CSHEI-enrolled districts raised

Table 7.1   General Statistics

	Colorado School Health Education Initiative Schools	Colorado Schools
Number of schools	156	1,568
Number of students	62,390	699,135
Number of teachers	3,605	37,840
Graduation rate	84%	80%
Per-pupil spending	$7,759	$7,036

Table 7.2   Student Ethnicity (percentages of total enrollment)

	Colorado School Health Education Initiative Schools	Colorado Schools
American Indian	2.5	1.2
Asian	1.1	2.7
Black	1.5	5.6
Hispanic	37.2	19.9
White	57.6	70.6

the per-pupil spending average for the group to above the state average. Overall, CSHEI districts enjoyed somewhat higher than average graduation rates. As a group, these districts served higher percentages of Hispanic and American Indian students, but lower percentages of White, Asian, and Black students, than did other school districts in Colorado.

In what follows, we examine the degree to which the districts' capacity for implementing, building, and sustaining school health education programs increased, and we describe the extent to which environments supportive of health education were created through, and as a result of, these activities.

The Outcomes of the Initiative

As we describe in this section, outcomes realized by CSHEI included the widespread review and adoption of research-based school health education programs, an increase in adequately trained teachers and other staff to teach adopted programs, the development of new school health education leaders to enhance the likelihood that comprehensive school health education would remain a part of the schools and their communities, and the effective use of

HEACs to increase the involvement of key individuals within the school and community, including parents, students, school administrators, and teachers.

DEVELOPING LOCAL LEADERS: HEALTH EDUCATION COORDINATOR GROWTH AND DEVELOPMENT

The professional growth and development that occurred among the 14 HECs is one of the most significant impacts of CSHEI. Through a combination of "real-world" experience, professional development activities, and technical assistance from RMC staff, the HECs demonstrated considerable growth throughout the initiative in several areas:

- Knowledge about comprehensive health education programs and models of coordinated school health

- Knowledge and awareness of health education programs and policies within coordinators' own districts and schools

- Skills as both project coordinators and HECs in areas such as managing project budgets, writing grants, and planning teacher training

- Building local support for school health and health education programs through HEACs, the publication of newsletters, meetings with administrators and teachers, and periodic updates to local school boards

- Gaining skills in data collection methods, interpretation, and report writing for evaluation

- Advocating for school health education through public speaking and with the use of local media

Figure 7.3 presents data on the self-reported confidence of HECs before and after their CSHEI experiences.

COMMUNITY TEAMWORK: REVIEWING, SELECTING, AND ADOPTING HEALTH EDUCATION CURRICULA

Throughout the course of a site's enrollment in CSHEI, an HEAC's core task was to select health education curricula for public review and to make recommendations to the school board based on public feedback, the review of local data, and internal committee discussions. Committee members also worked to develop or revise health education standards and policies supporting the teaching of health and, more generally, to support other efforts to build a coordinated school health education program. However, curricular review

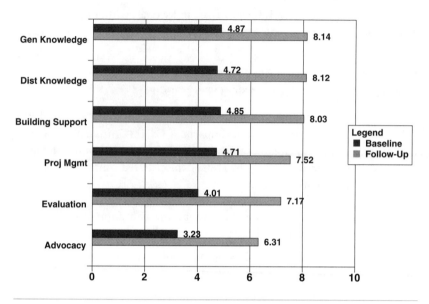

Figure 7.3   Increase in Capacity Among Health Education Coordinators

NOTE: The rating scales assessed HECs' own sense of how much confidence they had in carrying out various job-related tasks. Each rating was made using a Likert scale (from 0 to 10).

and selection remained the HEAC's primary responsibility. By the end of the initiative, nearly all districts (20 of 21) had reviewed, recommended, and adopted K–12 health education curricula.

As a result of their formation and these facilitated processes, HEACs achieved the following:

• Became school health education advocates, further enhancing the coordinators' role as local "champions" of health education

• Linked and supported key players in health education and health promotion/disease prevention so that local efforts and resources were expended in a complementary fashion rather than a redundant one

• Addressed other components of a coordinated school health program such as staff wellness, school counseling and support services, and family and community involvement in school health

• Raised awareness and increased knowledge of HEAC members about school health education

• Established priorities for sustaining CSHEI efforts, including the need for future funding and the continuation of the HEC position

Despite the fact that most members of the HEACs had a professional and/or personal interest in (school) health education, the largest percentage of respondents to our HEAC member self-report surveys ($N = 326$) reported the following impacts of committee participation:

• Increased knowledge about effective health education (96%)
• Increased commitment to school health education (93%)
• Increased awareness of issues surrounding health education (96%)
• Increased appreciation of challenges faced by teachers who implement school health education curricula (96%)

HEACs provided a forum for community members working and living in diverse settings to come together and learn about one another. For example, committee members from outside the school system reported that, as a result of their participation on the HEAC, they gained a greater appreciation for the challenges that teachers experience in implementing health education curricula. In many cases, according to interviews with stakeholders in the processes, HEACs worked more effectively than other school-related committees, and their reviews of health education curricula were often far more thorough than the reviews of curricula for other content areas.

By their own reports, members of the HEACs deemed the development and operation of their committees to have been a success. Broadly constituted, these committees consisted of members of their local communities and school districts. In their operations, these committees determined their own membership rules, operating norms, and decision-making processes. Three additional attributes contributed to their self-perceived success. First, formal and informal data collection about communities and students (e.g., needs, wants, assets) helped these committees to make informed decisions about curricula and other related health activities. Second, dedicated time for community and committee discussion permitted diverse perspectives to be heard and concerns to be addressed about particular curricula. Third, skilled facilitation (usually by the HEC but also by RMC staff and other committee members) made this deliberate attention to student needs and diverse community perspectives possible.

The overwhelming majority of HEAC survey respondents reported that they were satisfied with the processes used by the HEACs—a remarkable achievement given the diversity in committee membership and the relative sensitivity of the issues with which these committees often dealt. A large percentage of respondents were satisfied with the goals of the committees (89%), committee leadership (87%), the way in which decisions were made (79%), committee progress to date (77%), the clarity of missions and purposes (87%), and the clarity of decision making (79%). HEAC members believed that the technical assistance devoted to developing and sustaining effective processes within these committees enabled them to deal effectively with controversy. Although controversy occurred in some CSHEI districts, it tended not to derail the primary aim of selecting curricula because effective group processes were established, developed, and supported. In one district where controversy over health education was relatively pronounced, one committee member noted, "The HEAC works better together than other similar groups in the past . . . [when] there were breakdowns between parents and teachers. . . . [Now] there is less animosity among members." Another committee member added, "The HEAC leadership is an essential part of the process working well."

EXPERT TEACHERS: TEACHER
TRAINING IN ADOPTED CURRICULA

During CSHEI, approximately 1,300 elementary school staff members and 120 secondary school staff members attended initiative curricular training. In each CSHEI district, nearly every elementary school teacher and each secondary school health teacher received training at least once. Results of both training evaluations and elementary school teacher implementation surveys indicate that after attending CSHEI-sponsored training events, teachers felt adequately prepared to teach the adopted curriculum and confident that they could go back to the classroom and teach it to their students. Our analysis of 419 teacher surveys found that after training, 81% of teachers felt positive about the curriculum and 73% felt adequately prepared to teach the curriculum.

Increased Capacity Within Districts

CSHEI clearly left schools with more capacity to offer students more effective school health education programs and to develop other components of a coordinated health education program. This increased capacity can be measured in a variety of ways within local sites. In each CSHEI district, a variety of community members and school district representatives became active participants as well as skilled and knowledgeable advocates for school health education, as described in the HEAC survey results summarized previously. Effective processes for maintaining open constructive dialogue were established and sustained. Most districts reviewed and adopted sound, research-based health education curricula at all levels (elementary, middle, and high school) according to local priorities and values and had teachers trained to teach these effective programs. Other districts also created other, non-classroom-based health education programs such as staff wellness and counseling.

FROM ADOPTION TO IMPLEMENTATION

Despite CSHEI's success in building the capacity of HECs, HEACs, and teachers, implementation of the elementary school curricula was limited. Although we have emphasized the work of coordinators and advisory committees in carrying out CSHEI processes, the classroom teachers turned out to be the critical determinant of whether or not effective health education actually reached students and, therefore, whether or not CSHEI was likely to actually influence health, wellness, and disease. For elementary school teachers, this required not only learning a new curriculum but also finding ways in which to teach health along with other core content areas such as reading and math. Unfortunately, elementary school teachers taught less of the adopted curriculum than was anticipated, reflecting state and district pressures to devote increased attention to reading, writing, and math.

One year after CSHEI-related training, approximately 10% of teachers taught the entire adopted curriculum, with the majority (71%) teaching fewer than half of the lessons. Two years after the training, 81% of teachers were teaching fewer than half of the lessons. This trend is contrary to what was expected based on staff development research indicating that the longer teachers teach a curriculum, the more comfortable they become with it and the more likely they are to teach it. Examples of successful curriculum integration such as this are typically conducted under "ideal" conditions where there is sufficient classroom time for teaching health education and adequate resources for booster trainings and ongoing support. Findings from this initiative that more than 60% of teachers reported integrating health into other content areas and, on average, modified about half of the lessons reinforce what CSHEI teachers told us about the lack of classroom time for teaching health education—an obvious barrier to fuller curriculum implementation with fidelity.[2]

Despite the fact that CSHEI-funded districts officially adopted health education curricula and sent teachers to state-of-the-art training, teachers did not report teaching a large percentage of these adopted curricula to their students. Students in CSHEI sites, however, *were* more likely to be exposed to current or updated health education information through their receipt of some of these research-based curricula. Furthermore, the health education that elementary school students did receive was more likely a part of a comprehensive plan for health education, relevant to student needs and coordinated across grade levels, with most elementary school students in CSHEI districts scheduled to receive additional health education programming as they progressed into secondary school.

Implications for School Health Education
Program Planning and Implementation

State, regional, and local factors exerted strong influences over the success of school districts and individuals within them to review, discuss, recommend, train, and prepare for the implementation of health education curricula and programs. From our extensive interview and survey data from HECs, HEAC members, community members, teachers, district personnel, and others, we highlight a few strongly influential factors:

- Standards
- Funding
- District support systems
- Technical assistance

STANDARDS

Among all of the factors that influenced the CSHEI implementation experience, those at the state level were the most significant in determining the course of the actual classroom teaching of carefully selected health education curricula. In 1996, newly passed Colorado legislation mandated that all students would be tested in reading, writing, and math, beginning with elementary school students. The implications of the reform legislation were more fully realized in the fall of 1997 when regional and local newspapers published fourth-grade reading and writing test scores, putting public pressure on schools to address their apparent deficiencies in these content areas. As a result of the emphasis placed on reading, writing, and math by political officials and, consequently, by district administrators and teachers, much less time was available to commit to teaching health education (particularly in the elementary school grade levels, where a single classroom teacher is responsible for teaching all subject areas). One teacher in a CSHEI district explained, "I have used [the adopted curriculum] for the last 2 years, and I really enjoy it. I completely support health education. . . . Unfortunately, this past year . . ., I was required to teach reading, writing, and math and [to] put aside secondary subjects like health."

FUNDING

Money is a critical factor to building the capacity of school districts to select and implement effective health education curricula. The funds from CSHEI allowed districts to facilitate important communication among stakeholders, update curricular materials, train teachers, and hire coordinators to lead the entire process. Particularly as districts face pressure to focus on reading, writing, and math in the elementary school grades, a dedicated stream of funding for health education supported work that would not have happened otherwise.

On the other hand, the funding from The Colorado Trust, although generous, may not have been sufficient to produce the desired outcome of comprehensive school health education implemented throughout Grades K–12. Even though the health education coordinator typically laid a good foundation for implementation, it was not possible for one person to ensure that the curriculum was fully taught in every classroom. For that to happen, the district must commit its own financial resources as well.

Local funding becomes even more important over time. CSHEI presumed that the local districts would pick up the costs of the health education coordinator position to sustain the curriculum development work completed under the grants. However, not all districts honored that commitment, putting at risk the progress that had been made in the area of comprehensive health education.

DISTRICT SUPPORT SYSTEMS

As local newspaper accounts reveal, local community members can be influential in supporting or opposing health education in public schools. Although most of the respondents to our interviews and surveys acknowledged the *potential* for controversy surrounding the adoption of health education curricula, controversy either did not arise to the degree anticipated or failed to derail the process of adopting school health education programs. The relative inclusiveness of CSHEI processes, the fact that group norms and selection criteria were determined and agreed to collectively, and the presence of skilled facilitators (HECs and RMC staff) all contributed to an environment that tolerated disagreement but staved off conflict. Most districts (17 of 21) reported very little public controversy regarding the selection and adoption of health education curricula.

Similarly, district administrators and school boards play an influential role in whether health becomes an important curricular focus. Most school boards in the CSHEI districts were supportive of health education and officially adopted health education curricula for their districts. In contrast, principals and other district administrators (e.g., superintendents, curriculum directors) exerted both positive and negative influences over the implementation of health education curricula at both district and school building levels. Although the principals we interviewed viewed health education as important, it was frequently seen as less important than other content areas, namely reading, writing, and math. This often translated into ambivalent messages about how much health curriculum teachers were expected to teach. Our survey of more than 200 elementary school teachers in CSHEI districts in the spring of 1999 showed a drop in the number of lessons they thought their principals expected them to teach.

TECHNICAL ASSISTANCE

Technical assistance from RMC encompassed a wide variety of activities to a diverse array of recipients (Chavis & Florin, 1990). Although much of RMC's technical assistance supported the work of health education coordinators in school districts and communities, RMC staff viewed HECs as much more than coordinators and administrators of local programs, seeing these professionals as leaders and champions for health education at the local, regional, and state levels as well as critical linking agents between school districts and communities. In addition to providing ongoing professional development opportunities, RMC staff actively fostered the development of a health education coordinator network to expand the resource capacity of this group of professionals.

In addition to the ongoing professional development opportunities provided to HECs, RMC staff offered facilitation training to HEAC members and opened professional development opportunities to other community/district representatives. This support enhanced the capacity of local districts and communities to advance the cause of school health education. RMC also compiled timely accurate information to key stakeholders concerning current research on health education curricula, opportunities for professional development and training, and additional funding opportunities to enhance school health education efforts. In addition, RMC staff provided technical assistance and support to those sites that chose to undertake local evaluation efforts. One HEC commented on the timely assistance: "In every endeavor I undertook, I had advice and support from the RMC staff. They would touch base with me throughout my experiences, and many times they would supply information before I even knew I had questions."

At the regional, state, and national levels, RMC staff served as linking agents to many other organizations and agencies that could provide information and other forms of technical assistance as needed. CSHEI districts further benefited from the fact that RMC was accessible through a toll-free telephone number, a newsletter, and a Web site.

Conclusions

CSHEI was designed to develop the capacity of schools to implement and sustain effective comprehensive school health education programs. By establishing mechanisms to help schools develop and improve school health programs through HECs and HEACs, the initiative provided schools and districts with the capacity to offer students more effective school health education programs and to develop other components of a coordinated health education program. Benefits that participating districts and schools have realized include the following:

- Research-based curricula
- Resource materials
- Trained teachers
- People within the district and the community who support school health education programs
- Skilled and knowledgeable district staff (the HECs and HEAC members)
- Models for effective, informed, participatory decision making (the HEACs)
- Some additional health education components (e.g., staff wellness, counseling)

Despite these significant changes in capacity, however, we found that elementary school students in CSHEI districts were not getting as much exposure to effective health education programs as was intended by the initiative. CSHEI began just when state and local pressures for improved standardized test scores in Colorado became an overriding priority. This academic climate created a new set of pressures on elementary school teachers and resulted in core subject areas, such as reading and math, taking curricular time away from the newly adopted health education programs. Consequently, the initiative had limited effects on the *implementation* of research-based comprehensive health education curricula at the elementary school level.

At the community and district levels, CSHEI succeeded in developing the capacity of individuals and districts to "create and enhance" effective school health education programs. In accordance with the literature and "best practices," the initiative developed local leaders, created effective committees to review and recommend health education curricula and programs, trained teachers, and raised awareness about health and health education. Even where there was local controversy, these coordinators and committees moved ahead effectively in their discussions and decisions around health education. Unfortunately, one of the greatest barriers to the implementation of selected curricula was the shift in Colorado education focus and policies. This created an emphasis on statewide improvements in reading, writing, and math test scores at the critical point when most CSHEI schools were beginning to implement their chosen health education curricula. To date, the districts throughout the Colorado school system continue to emphasize test scores in core content subjects (reading, writing, and math) as the primary criterion of school performance.

The CSHEI evaluation findings provide valuable information about the realities of how school health education curricula are adopted and implemented in schools. These results reinforce the importance of paying attention to the "social ecology" of schools and the need to develop district capacity at many levels within the school and community. The CSHEI experience highlights the following strategic building blocks necessary to enhance the implementation of comprehensive school health education in local schools:

- A community climate that values health education in schools

- Leadership from within schools and school boards that views health education as an essential part of every student's K–12 educational experience

- Teachers who are adequately trained in effective health education programs and practices

- The coordination of school and community-based programs so that youth are exposed to health education in a variety of settings

- Effective (i.e., research-based) K–12 school health education programs

- The integration of school health education with other subject areas

- Clear expectations of what and how much K–12 health education should be taught

Within the CSHEI, all of these components were in place except the last two. It remains to be seen whether the professional capacity development realized in the participating districts will be translated into further health education program efforts in the future.

Notes

1. CSHEI staff did not require a formal grant proposal as part of the application process. Rather, they requested that each potential site develop a school district/community profile.

2. Once 1-year implementation data were disseminated, (a) implementation became a discussion topic at nearly every HEC meeting, (b) RMC provided additional training and resources for enhancing curricular integration, and (c) RMC offered booster or follow-up trainings but did not strongly encourage or require them. These efforts, however, did not slow or reverse decrements in implementation.

References

Allensworth, D. D., Lawson, E., Nicholson, L., & Wyche, J. H. (Eds.). (1997). *Schools and health: Our nation's investment*. Washington, DC: National Academy Press.

Bracht, N. F. (1990). *Health promotion at the community level*. Newbury Park, CA: Sage.

Centers for Disease Control and Prevention. (1998). *Youth risk behavior survey: Youth97* [CD-ROM]. Atlanta, GA: Author.

Centers for Disease Control and Prevention. (2000). *Leading causes of mortality and morbidity and contributing behaviors by state, 1999 (United States)*. [Online]. Retrieved September 11, 2000, from the World Wide Web: www.cdc.gov/nccdphp/dash/yrbs/pies99/natl.htm

Centers for Disease Control and Prevention. (2001). *School health programs: An investment in our nation's future*. Atlanta, GA: Author.

Chavis, D. M., & Florin, P. (1990). Nurturing grassroots initiatives for health and housing. *Bulletin of the New York Academy of Medicine, 66,* 558–572.

Collins, J. L., Small, M. L., Kann, L., Pateman, B. C., Gold, R. S., & Kolbe, L. J. (1995). School health education. *Journal of School Health, 65,* 302–311.

Dusenbury, L., & Falco, M. (1995). Eleven components of effective drug abuse prevention curricula. *Journal of School Health, 65,* 420–425.

Dusenbury, L., & Lake, A. (1996). *Making the grade: A guide to school drug prevention programs.* Washington, DC: Drug Strategies.

Joint Committee on National Health Education Standards. (1995). *Achieving health literacy: An investment in the future.* Atlanta, GA: American Cancer Society.

Joyce, B., & Showers, B. (1995). *Student achievement through staff development: Fundamentals of school renewal.* White Plains, NY: Longman.

Kirby, D. (1997). *No easy answers: Research findings on programs to reduce teen pregnancy.* Washington, DC: National Campaign to Prevent Teen Pregnancy.

Lohrmann, D. K., & Wooley, S. F. (1998). Comprehensive school health education. In E. Marx, S. Wooley, & D. Northrop (Eds.), *Health is academic: A guide to coordinated school health programs.* New York: Teachers College Press.

Marx, E., Wooley, S., & Northrop, D. (Eds.) (1998). *Health is academic: A guide to coordinated school health programs.* New York: Teachers College Press.

National Center for Health Statistics. (1999). *Healthy People 2000 review, 1998–99.* Hyattsville, MD: Public Health Service.

Prochaska, J. O., & DiClemente, C. C. (1984). *The transtheoretical approach: Crossing traditional boundaries of change.* Homewood, IL: Dow Jones–Irwin.

Resnicow, K., & Allensworth, D. D. (1996). Conducting a comprehensive school health program. *Journal of School Health, 66,* 59–63.

8

Home Visitation Learning Groups

Community-Based Professionals Discovering Best Practices

Thomas I. Miller

Michelle Miller Kobayashi

Peggy L. Hill

Bringing together service providers within a learning group setting represents a novel and potentially enriching opportunity to allow the group's participants to increase their professional skills, to network with their peers both within and outside their communities, and to develop common goals for client service delivery. In this chapter, case study information is presented on five such groups formed in Colorado between 1998 and 2000, specifically to promote learning opportunities related to the delivery of home visitation services.

As described in this chapter, the unique feature of the learning group approach from the perspective of community-based health promotion lies in the interaction it promotes between the service provider community and the clients these providers collectively work to serve. Although the directions and activities of the learning groups formed in Colorado have been found to be distinctly idiosyncratic, in their optimally realized form, learning groups offer the following array of benefits to improved community health:

- The opportunity for home visitation service providers to improve their knowledge of peers providing similar services in other agencies

- Structured settings in which home visitation professionals can individually and collectively consider options for improving the ways in which services are delivered to clients

- The opportunity to gain information on "best practices" models and ways in which to measure service delivery effectiveness

The evaluation results of this intervention show that with limited initial funding ($5,000 per year per community over 2 years), the participating learning group members invested a substantial amount of volunteer time (6,930 hours) and achieved 98% of their originally proposed goals. The findings further suggest that the potential benefits of the learning group model can be enhanced through attention to the development of a common group vision, careful selection of the project facilitator, increased funding, and more targeted attention to improvements in client service delivery. Given the accomplishments of the learning groups described in this chapter, this approach would appear to offer substantial benefits to other types of professional groups and service providers that are interested in using a "learning" model for improving the delivery of services to clients they are mutually interested in serving.

What Is Home Visitation and What Are Learning Groups?

The vision for the project was to develop the capacity of individuals and organizations delivering home visitation services in Colorado to use research literature, program evaluation, and critical reflection on practice as tools for program planning and program improvement. Home visitation is a service delivery strategy that provides resources to people in their homes. In the context of the learning groups project, home visitation programs are designed to work primarily with young families, to whom staff (professional, paraprofessional, or volunteer) provide home-based support and guidance of different types and at varying levels of intensity and duration, typically centered on perinatal and newborn care. Communities in Colorado currently support more than 100 home visiting programs, each of which operates with a set of beliefs about what works best to meet the varied needs of the families it serves.

All service programs, including home visiting agencies, can benefit from being engaged in a continual process of reflection on their existing practices and from an evaluation of their program effectiveness. The premise behind the Home Visitation Learning Groups (HVLG) initiative has been that this reflection process should be regular, provocative, and supportive, guiding participants toward knowledge about programs that have been found to be effective and encouraging them to adopt practices that hold real promise of serving families better.

In the HVLG initiative, a *learning group* has been defined as "a cluster of home visiting program directors and staff who work together in an ongoing facilitated process of reflection on practice and program improvement." The primary goals of this learning group pilot project were to (a) enhance learning and promote organizational change and (b) improve home visitation services for at-risk families with young children. Having groups come together on a voluntary basis, define their own questions, and assume responsibility for their own learning was thought to facilitate a more user-friendly approach to learning as compared with more traditional, didactic teaching methods.

Learning groups were designed to provide an opportunity for the participating individuals to improve the home visitor programs they were representing. Service providers and program managers rarely have the opportunity to engage in a reflective process of developing and refining the logic of the work they do with their clients, let alone to receive the type of support and "friendly challenge" that allows them to improve their approach.

The following features were included in the learning group model to help participants integrate new knowledge into their work as program managers and practitioners: (a) exercises that prodded participants to articulate the theory and logic that formed the basis for their programs, (b) a review of mechanisms for evaluating the quality of implementation and effectiveness of participants' current program practices, and (c) the freedom and support to make desired program changes. In setting up this approach, the HVLG initiative assumed that the development of a clear program logic that is solidly grounded in well-tested theory is an essential step for any community-based program interested in enhancing program quality. Program logic becomes the guide for initial program design, for program evaluation, for continued examination of relevant literature, and for reflection on clinical experience and program improvement. The learning groups were designed in such a way that participants helped one another (and held each other accountable) in developing a well-articulated program logic, in increasing the underlying knowledge base of home visitation research, and in improving programs. Through these mechanisms, learning groups were designed to provide a means for the participating programs to become more effective in serving families and to develop a clearer, more rigorous framework to guide their future program development efforts.

Although much of the initial focus of the project was on individual and group learning, opportunities also existed for the groups to consider collective ways in which home visiting agencies could work together to meet their clients' needs in a more efficient, coherent fashion. At the same time that the members of a learning group were examining the logic and effectiveness of their own programs, they might also look at the larger picture to see whether the mix of services currently available to local residents was "comprehensive" (in terms of who was being served and the mix of services available). Thus, learning groups also provided a means for the expansion and/or coordination of home visitation services within the participating communities.

The HVLG initiative also had a broader goal of establishing a grassroots learning network of practitioners dedicated to (a) keeping their programs on the cutting edge of the home visitation knowledge base and (b) deepening their understanding about what does and does not work in the challenging business of strengthening families. As home visitation programs improved their effectiveness, and as home visitation practitioners developed a more reflective, data-driven approach to program development, it was hoped that home visitation in Colorado would gain credibility as a legitimate means of improving child and maternal outcomes, thereby increasing the base of financial support from government agencies and private grant makers.

Finally, it should be noted that the HVLG initiative was set up as a pilot project. The Colorado Trust was interested in whether the learning groups model could be successfully implemented with informal coalitions of home visitation programs from diverse regions of Colorado. If so, the next question is whether this learning approach can be replicated in other home visitation settings and also in other health and human service domains.

How Was the Program Evaluated?

The evaluation of the HVLG project consisted of three primary components: (a) review of the progress reports and other documents prepared by the learning groups; (b) telephone interviews with program participants, facilitators, and the program director; and (c) a retreat where focused discussions were held with learning group participants. In addition, evaluators traveled to southern Colorado to conduct discussions with the Montezuma County participants who could not attend the larger retreat.

An interim evaluation was also performed midway through the study by the project's executive director. Numerous important results from this study were used for midcourse improvements to several of the learning groups. As examples, one learning group received money for program improvements that had been initially targeted, but not spent, for facilitator time. Another group determined that it needed to change its facilitator. Several other projects were able to move from learning to doing, receiving support for next phase proposals. The interim findings were also used to provide information on each group's developmental process and to focus areas for the final evaluation.

How Did This Program Begin and What Makes It Community Based?

Starting in 1993, The Colorado Trust funded the Home Visitation 2000 initiative, a large-scale, randomized clinical trial to test the effectiveness of nurse and paraprofessional home visitation early in the life cycle (Olds & Hill, 1998). As an extension of the research on home visitation outcomes, the Prevention Research Center for Family and Child Health obtained funding to convene groups of home visitation professionals for the purpose of self-directed learning. This learning was to be based on "the participants' reflection on practice, on relevant research literature, [and on] their own direct experience with families" (Olds & Hill, 1998, p. 1), and the learning was expected to result in program improvement. In announcing the availability of funds for the learning groups, the request for proposals (RFP) stated, "The result of each Learning Group's work should enhance the quality of home visiting programs and contribute to a community's efforts to support healthy family development."

The RFP elicited proposals from 14 groups of home visitation practitioners from communities throughout Colorado, and The Colorado Trust awarded funding to 5 of these applicant groups in March 1998. The foundation provided each group with $5,000 per year in grant funds over a 24-month period and paid for an outside facilitator, selected by the group, who would spend up to 20 days per year serving the group. Each group was responsible for identifying its own members, specifying its own learning goals, and determining the best methods for reaching its goals.

In all, the five learning groups consisted of 30 agencies and roughly 47 participants. A typical learning group consisted of 5 to 7 agencies and had approximately 9 members. The Mesa County Learning Group was unique in that it involved just 1 agency: the Mesa County Health Department. Although some agencies specialized entirely in home visitation services, many were responsible for providing other health and human services to their communities. A brief description of the five learning groups follows in the next section.

The Five Learning Groups

MESA COUNTY LEARNING GROUP

Group Composition

The Mesa County Learning Group was formed by the home visitation public health nurses of the Mesa County Health Department. Nine service providers participated in the group over the grant period. The group met approximately 37 times in addition to the kickoff retreat and mid-grant evaluation. Collectively, participants reported spending approximately 1,850 hours over the 24 months working on the grant, including group meeting times and the time spent between meetings preparing for the discussions.

Learning Group Goals

The original and evolving goals developed by the Mesa County Learning Group were as follows:

- Formalize a process for public health nursing home visitation that increases effectiveness in identifying and enhancing family strengths to improve family health outcomes for high-risk families of Mesa County. (Capture a fluid process that embodies the best practices of public health nurse home visitation, regardless of the specific program.)

- Facilitate the ability of home visitors to mentor senior nursing students from Mesa State College during their community health rotation.

- Identify the target population.

- Explore, identify, and select/develop assessment tools to use with families at intake, as well as periodically throughout the intervention process, to determine progress.

- Explore, identify, and select/develop an intervention model.

- Improve health outcomes of the families served by more effective assessment, diagnosis, planning, implementation, and evaluation.

- Be able to reach more families, decrease noncompliance and failed visits, empower families to make healthy changes, and thereby effect significant change in the community's health.

- Increase job satisfaction, building a strong team.

Group Activities and Outcomes

During the grant period, the following activities were undertaken by the Mesa County Learning Group:

- Developed a logic model (conceptual framework)
- Surveyed group members and other staff on training needs and what they want from an assessment tool/charting information
- Took the Meyers-Briggs psychological profiling test and debriefed the results
- Designed a Family Information Form (including drafting, revising, piloting, etc.)
- Designed a Client Contact Form (including drafting, revising, piloting, etc.)
- Purchased and implemented computer software and hardware for assessment/ evaluation
- Began designing additional topic-specific assessment forms
- Held workshops or in-services on various continuing education topics

MONTEZUMA COUNTY LEARNING GROUP

Group Composition

Six home visitation programs participated in the Montezuma County Learning Group. The group met about once each month during the 2-year grant period. During this time, participants reported spending 810 hours as a group working on the grant.

Learning Group Goals

In general, the Montezuma County Learning Group goals related to gaining greater coordination and networking among programs providing home visitation services as well as to gaining more knowledge about specific types of training, research, and evaluation options.

Group Activities and Outcomes

During the grant period, the following activities were undertaken by the Montezuma County Learning Group:

- Attended home visitation and fatherhood conferences
- Developed a list of traits needed for successful work with clients
- Reviewed background material on the Home Visitation 2000 model and developed a preliminary logic model listing common program objectives
- Held a Cultural Diversity Panel
- Hosted presentations from the Department of Social Services regarding the Child Health Plan and from Child Protection Services

- Hosted workshops on child abuse and neglect, interviewing, adult learning skills, reflective supervision, parent-infant interaction, and infant brain development
- Developed a referral form to allow greater collaboration among participating agencies
- Reviewed how each program works, where referrals come from, and what is done on first and subsequent visits
- Discussed making service coordination workable for a family and promoting functional outcomes in natural environments

SUMMIT COUNTY LEARNING GROUP

Group Composition

The Summit County Learning Group was initiated by a local doctor, who was joined by directors, coordinators, supervisors, and volunteers representing five agencies serving Summit County. Eleven programs ultimately participated in the learning group, each of which served families in the community through some form of home visitation. The timing of home visitation provided by each agency varied, with some conducting these visits during the prenatal period, others visiting mothers soon after birth, and the remainder visiting homes with children from ages 3 months to 3 years. The populations served by these home visitation programs also differed. Some home visitors focused their services on families with infants and toddlers at risk for developmental problems, others addressed families at risk for child abuse or neglect, and several others offered their services to all families in the community. Participants reported spending more than 1,500 hours as a group over the grant period.

Learning Group Goals

In its original proposal, the Summit County Learning Group included goals related to three topic areas: service coordination, finding additional funding sources, and learning more about and implementing quality evaluation. After meeting together for a while and making progress on these goals, the group added a fourth goal: identifying the gaps in home visitation services and finding ways in which to meet these needs.

Group Activities and Outcomes

During the grant period, the Summit County Learning Group undertook the following activities:

- Reviewed home visitation curricula, articles on evaluation, and other relevant materials
- Completed a matrix of services
- Completed a program logic model
- Began working on the Healthy Start Network
- Participated in numerous trust-building activities
- Applied for and received outside funding for programs
- Participated in a number of values clarification activities related to participant beliefs and philosophy related to family services
- Held an all-day learning group retreat

WESTERN SLOPE LEARNING GROUP

Group Composition

The Western Slope Learning Group began with the directors, coordinators, or supervisors from five agencies serving seven counties in western Colorado. Each program served families in the community through some form of home visitation. The home visitation program models represented included Parents as Teachers, Healthy Families America, Resource Mothers, and neighbor-to-neighbor/parent-to-parent programs. Populations served by these participating groups included families with infants and toddlers at risk for developmental problems, families at risk for child abuse or neglect, healthy families with infants and toddlers, and families with children up to 18 years of age. The group met approximately 16 times in addition to the kickoff retreat and reported spending more than 1,490 collective hours over the grant period. The group also hosted two conferences and participated in group conference calls.

Learning Group Goals

As with many of the groups, the Western Slope Learning Group set a large number of goals related to improving group cohesion and networking; sharing program materials, exploring new curriculum, and refining their own programs; identifying evaluation tools and learning how to use them; and exploring issues of staff training and supervision.

Group Activities and Outcomes

During the grant period, the Western Slope Learning Group undertook the following activities:

- Reviewed home visitation curricula from each other's agencies as well as national parenting and child development curricula

- Discussed cultural perspectives to improve client services
- Created program logic models for each agency and compared individual program logic models within the learning group to find common program goals and impacts
- Created cross-agency program logic models for topics such as family management skills, emotional support, and identifying strengths
- Toured each other's facilities
- Found common denominators in data collected in each agency and explored ways in which to use this information
- Hosted a statewide conference on home visitation and a Western Slope Learning Group conference for agency home visitation staff, inviting the Montezuma County Learning Group to participate
- Explored the role of evaluation in home visitation and studied effective models of evaluation in home visitation
- Networked with each other and with members of other learning groups
- Continuously examined group goals, accomplishments to date, and the role of the facilitator in the learning group

DENVER LEARNING GROUP

Group Composition

The Denver Learning Group consisted of the coordinators of seven programs in the Denver metro area. Each program served families at risk for child abuse and neglect through some form of home visitation component. The method of home visitation provided by each agency varied (e.g., Parents as Teachers, Visitantes, Family Advocates), as did the populations served (e.g., Hispanic/Latino, African American, Caucasian). The coordinators from the seven agencies had met during the year prior to the grant to share resources and coordinate activities. Participants reported spending more than 1,288 hours as a group over the 23 to 24 months working on grant activities. These time estimates included group meeting times and the time spent between meetings preparing for the discussions.

Learning Group Goals

The Denver Learning Group held four primary goals: learning about the full range of home visitation services, learning about evaluation tools, learning how the logic model can be applied to improve programs, and learning to engage families in a positive process. A year into the grant, the learning group decided to refocus its goals on learning about and developing outcome tools for home visitation and family advocacy. Group members were also interested in learning how to present evaluation results to funders effectively. Goals changed for a number of reasons, including changes in group membership and facilitation, the refinement of priorities, and the feeling that other baseline goals had already been met.

Group Activities and Outcomes

During the grant period, the following activities were undertaken by the Denver Learning Group:

- Review of home visitation practices
- Discussion of cultural perspectives to improve client services
- Creation of an activity grid presenting services offered by learning group agencies
- Study of the "theories of change" model
- Development of a preliminary draft of a logic model
- The attendance by four group members at a home visitation conference in Atlanta, Georgia, that had an evaluation emphasis

The Denver Learning Group disbanded 18 months into the grant cycle. Denver's urban setting, with its rich and complex mix of social service programs, seems to have been one important factor in limiting the success of the learning group. The incentives against participating in the group may have exceeded the benefits afforded by the initiative—limited financial support and the potential for learning and linking together to coordinate services. In addition, the Denver project was challenged by the early departure of the grant writer.

Study Findings

LEARNING GROUP OUTCOMES

To determine the participants' overall opinions regarding the benefits they derived from participating in the HVLG project, a survey was conducted that presented project participants with a list of potential outcomes or results of the learning group activities and asked them to what extent their knowledge, attitudes, or behavior had changed in specific areas as a result of the experience.

The degree to which participants increased their knowledge is shown in Figure 8.1. More than 60% reported that they had changed "a lot" in their knowledge of the work of staff in other agencies. More than 40% reported "a

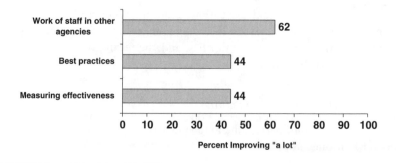

Figure 8.1   Learning Group Outcomes: Knowledge Changes

lot" of improvement in the areas of what works best in home visitation and measuring effectiveness.

In terms of attitudinal changes, a majority of participants reported that their attitudes had improved "a lot" in the areas of appreciation for other agency staff, increasing their sense of the importance of home visitation, and increasing their sense of the importance of learning (Figure 8.2). About 40% reported that they had improved "a lot" in their sense of their own abilities to serve clients. A smaller percentage of participants reported improvement in their willingness to spend time learning and in their concern over

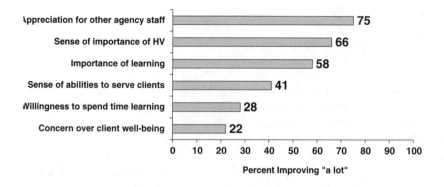

Figure 8.2   Learning Group Outcomes: Attitude Changes

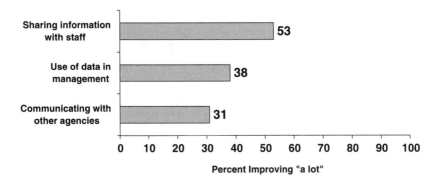

Figure 8.3   Learning Group Outcomes: Behavior Changes

client well-being. (Because the participants were very committed to both goals at the start of the project, it was difficult to observe changes in these areas.)

Relative to behavior changes, a majority of participants reported in the survey that they had improved "a lot" in the area of sharing information with staff within and outside their agencies (Figure 8.3). Nearly 40% said that they had increased their use of data "a lot" to help manage clients as a result of the HVLG project, and about 30% reported spending "a lot" more time communicating with staff from other agencies.

When asked in the focus groups whether they are now serving clients better because of the learning group experience, all of the groups said yes. Table 8.1 shows a number of specific ways in which each of the groups believed that it had improved its client services.

SUCCESSES

As described in the previous section, the five learning groups were unique in their specific goals and activities while sharing a common goal of working together to improve the delivery of home visitation services to their clients. Although the initial goals proposed by each learning group were ambitious, staff reported that more than 98% of the proposed goals were at least partially accomplished. The success of the groups may be attributed to the large amount of voluntary time committed to this project by most of the participants. On average, the time volunteered by participants in each individual group totaled approximately 1,400 total hours over the 24-month period. Across the entire

Table 8.1   Reported Improvements in Client Services

Mesa	Montezuma	Summit	Western Slope	Denver
• We learned to better identify client needs. • We are better prepared for visits. • Our work is appreciated by other agencies. • The knowledge gained has spilled over into other groups or projects.	• Families are getting more support. • We have increased recognition of what's out there. • With the use of evaluation tools, staff get the information they need to provide more focused assistance to families. • Coordination is smoother, even when using services within the health department.	• Learning allowed us to have the best program possible. • It's a better product if it's based on learning, research, etc. • We understand the need for ongoing learning and evaluation.	• The learning group helped me with my supervision of case visitors. • Our evaluation tools now are more family friendly. • My assessment of families is now based on strengths and assets, not needs. • I'm rejuvenated and revitalized.	• The cultural talk was useful in providing services to clients from other ethnic backgrounds. • The strengthening of relationships was key because the State of Colorado is requiring four of the agencies to come together to serve clients in the future. • The project was instrumental in getting the agencies to work together. Service will improve citywide and for new clients.

learning group project, 6,390 hours were committed to this effort. This rather large contribution of time and energy is even more impressive considering that each group was initially given only $10,000 plus facilitator time over the grant period. The devotion of the participants to the project speaks not only to the dedication of home visitation service providers but also to the importance of the work being done by the learning groups themselves.

Nearly all of the project's participants indicated that they would recommend the project to other providers and believed that the learning group experience was a worthwhile investment for the funders. When asked how they would convince funders to divert funds from direct service provision to the creation of learning groups, participants suggested that the learning groups approach is a long-term investment in creating a better product that will benefit all clients in the future. One learning group member summarized the importance of this long-term perspective as follows: "If you keep fetching bodies from the river and never investigate what's happening upstream, you won't be very effective."

The accomplishments of three of the learning groups have extended beyond the grant period with follow-on funding provided by The Colorado Trust. Groups are now working on the following:

- Implementing a new home visitation model
- Completing assessment and evaluation systems for home visitation
- Improving teamwork and transitioning toward a single service provider
- Making changes in other work arenas based on what was learned during the HVLG project

SUCCESSFUL TRAITS OF LEARNING GROUPS

Case studies of these five different learning groups help to provide insight regarding those aspects of the HVLG project that made for success and those that distracted from the learning goals of the individual groups. Factors contributing to group success are discussed in the following subsections.

Facilitators Well Matched to the Learning Groups

The facilitator played a key role in all of the learning groups and was extolled in groups where success was achieved and faulted in the groups where less was accomplished. The facilitators working with the groups varied in their knowledge bases and facilitation approaches, with no clear facilitator profile best fitting all learning groups. Attempts were made to assist each group in interviewing and selecting its own facilitator, but groups were allowed little time for this process, and some were not clear about their facilitation needs early in the project. As the project evolved, the facilitator traits considered to be important by all groups were flexibility, fairness, and the ability to share a common vision regarding where the group should progress over the grant period. Facilitators with content-relevant experience in either home visitation or evaluation were perceived as being able to move groups toward their goals more quickly.

A Common Vision and Shared Goals

The learning groups that held a common vision and shared goals for their projects from the onset reported achieving the greatest success. These groups were able to begin work immediately on intended outcomes and found the information presented and discussed in the groups regarding home visitation models to be relevant and important. Groups with a shared vision also had an easier time in transitioning between goals and in refocusing their efforts as their projects moved forward in time.

Group Composition Based on Cohesive Programs

The cohesiveness of the programs that comprised the learning groups influenced success as well. The groups that had worked together prior to the learning venture had more opportunity to develop clear operating goals and did better than groups that were more heterogeneous in terms of deciding what goals to pursue.

Commitment to Long-Term Gains and the Necessity of Short-Term Outcomes

The most successful groups were able to sustain their enthusiasm for the project because they were able to make short-term gains along the way. When asked how she stayed motivated to provide so much time for so little financial reimbursement, one participant responded, "I was trapped by the goodness of it." The recognition of short-term gains, coupled with the promise of long-term outcomes, was important enough to sustain the members.

The networking and social support from others within their field was immediately gratifying to many participants. These short-term gains may have been easier to realize for groups in less densely populated areas, where providers were more isolated and so had less regular access to a network of support.

CHALLENGES AND RECOMMENDATIONS

Although the learning group model, as applied in this pilot study, was by and large successful, the self-reported experience of the participants suggests that certain challenges were faced that in turn lend themselves to the following refinements to the model.

1. Creating uniform goals accepted by the varying agencies that comprise a learning group was identified as an important component of success. The absence of consensus, in turn, was found to be a predictor of a lower level of group activity and accomplishments. Similar to other community-based efforts, the presence of a strong sense of common purpose allowed groups to set aside individual allegiances and conflicts and enabled the learning groups to achieve their goals (Kreuter, Lezin, & Young, 2000). Incorporating a planning or "formative" phase could help some groups to begin the learning process with a shared vision.

2. Matching the facilitator to the learning group participants' needs and sensibilities was deemed an important aspect of success. Learning groups that are likely to survive conflicts, such as differences in project philosophies, need to be led by people who are seen as democratic and have strong conflict resolution, communication, and administrative skills (Kumpfer, Turner, Hopkins, & Librett, 1993). Allowing groups to become clearer about their needs during a planning or formative phase could increase the likelihood that a facilitator will be well matched to the group's expectations and goals.

3. The facilitators also provided an opportunity for linking learning groups together, if only through shared communication. Participants mentioned that this opportunity could have been used to greater advantage because each learning group seemed to operate in isolation from the others. Facilitators, as well as the project director, can become the linchpin to connecting various learning groups by increasing communications and interaction with other groups and then feeding back information to their members (Figure 8.4).

4. In managing an HVLG initiative (from the macro level), it is important that the project director be viewed as a "champion" for the learning groups process. Among other things, this means that the project director must be committed (and perceived as committed) to helping each learning group succeed in improving the effectiveness of the models that are represented in the group; in other words, groups need to be able to define success *on their own terms*. Although the executive director for the HVLG project was widely revered by virtually all learning group participants, there was some concern among participants and facilitators that, because of her institutional affiliation, the initiative might have an underlying agenda at odds with the learning group's philosophy. In particular, her connections to a study of the David Olds model of home visitation (Korfmacher, O'Brien, Hiatt, & Olds, 1999; Olds et al., 1997) suggested to some that the initiative was intended to displace existing community-based

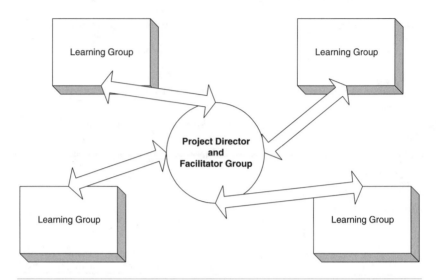

Figure 8.4   Networking Among Learning Groups

home visitation programs with that particular model. In future learning group grants, it may be prudent to find a way to separate more clearly the practices of a director from the expectations for the learning groups. Although every effort was made to disentangle the purpose of the learning groups from the specific model of home visitation in which the director had been involved, the effort was not a complete success. Creating an advisory board composed of practitioners or researchers associated with a variety of models who would present their models early in the project and remain as advisers throughout the project would serve three useful purposes: (a) expanding the array of home visitation models considered, (b) enhancing learning of best practices, and (c) affirming the message and providing the opportunity for technical assistance to demonstrate that a variety of home visitation models have credibility within the overall project.

5. Although four of the five groups were able to achieve significant results with the small amount of grant money made available, the time spent away from clients and direct service provision was a struggle for most participants. Because the home visitation providers were already challenged to meet the needs of their client base, some perceived that the time spent on learning impeded their immediate ability to provide a continuing level and quality of services to their clients.

Because of the great amount of work required of the learning group participants, the large distances traveled, and the considerable administrative work required, funders in the future may consider increasing the size of the learning group grants to ensure that costs can be fully covered for travel, use of administrative assistants, and coverage for staff during the time that they are to attend meetings. Studies of similar community-based projects suggest that group members must feel that the benefits of group membership outweigh the costs, a balance that in turn helps to reduce turnover and to maintain project momentum (Chinman, Anderson, & Imm, 1996; Gray, 1991).

6. Compressing the learning process is one other way in which to maintain project momentum. The RFP indicated that grants could last for "up to 24 months," but most participants took this to mean that the projects *were required* to last 24 months. It appears that in most cases, the same amount of learning and supporting activities could have been accomplished in 18 months, making it easier to sustain the enthusiasm necessary to maintain active participation.

7. At the heart of the HVLG initiative, there is a strong and reasonable presumption that improved learning by clinicians and staff will lead to better services to home-visited clients and, therefore, to healthier mothers, families, and children. Most of the work by learning group members, therefore, has been directed toward improving staff knowledge and practice. The focus of content learning on participating clinicians and staff rather than on changing the ways in which they provide services to clients meant that client services and client change remained a less direct area for program improvement. Although there is some research suggesting that it is more realistic for coalitions to focus initially on affecting policy and structural/environmental factors than on individual health outcomes (Kreuter et al., 2000), future funders may wish to augment the learning group experience by continuing to support these groups until their impacts can be measured at the client level. As the expansion of the learning groups model is considered, it may be helpful to broaden the focus to include, in the bull's eye of targeted outcomes, changes that staff learning create in client services and, ultimately, in client outcomes (Figure 8.5).

To respond to these challenges that emerged over the course of the HVLG initiative, we would recommend that the learning groups approach be structured in a way that establishes clearer expectations and that explicitly ties the learning process to the work that agencies are doing in the areas of program development and evaluation. More specifically, we would recommend that learning groups operate according to the model depicted in Figure 8.6. This model incorporates several changes that grow from our evaluation:

- Taking time in a planning process to learn about learning group participants and to create a set of uniform goals,
- Testing and hiring a facilitator,
- Using the learning period to focus on intended changes in service delivery and client outcomes

PURPOSE OF THE HOME
VISITATION LEARNING GROUP
INITIATIVE

RECOMMENDED APPROACH
TO ESTABLISHING A PURPOSE
FOR LEARNING GROUPS

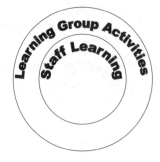

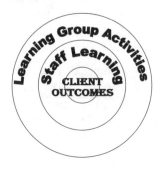

Figure 8.5   Grounding Learning Groups in a More Intrinsically Meaningful
Purpose

- Abbreviating the learning period to 18 months from 24
- Following a learning period with a period of implementation that will lead to better client outcomes and that would be supported with additional, and higher levels, of funding, and
- Incorporating process and outcome evaluation throughout the project's life.

Conclusions

Although unique in their specific goals, all five learning groups focused on the improvement of their home visitation services to clients. The more concrete activities of the groups included developing capacity grids that outlined the services being provided in the community and identified gaps in services, learning about the best practices for home visitation, hosting and attending conferences and seminars, creating logic models to describe service provision and desired outcomes, and developing outcome assessment tools.

The less tangible accomplishments included improved group communication and strengthened cohesion, increased professionalism, team building, improved conflict resolution skills, and a general rejuvenation of enthusiasm for work. The social support and networking was very important for providers, especially those practicing in the less urbanized areas of the state.

Can this learning approach be used in other health and social service settings? The evaluation results suggest that learning groups can benefit community health by focusing clinicians and administrators on best practices that ultimately improve client outcomes. Furthermore, this reflective time seems to enhance staff satisfaction and interagency networking, helping to attract and retain competent

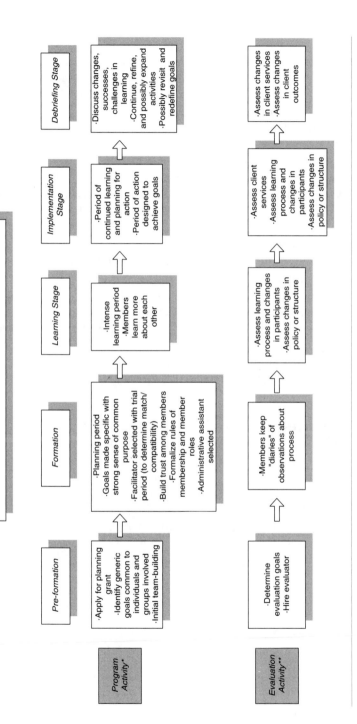

Model for Ideal Learning Group Process
to link learning and practice

| *Pre-formation* | *Formation* | *Learning Stage* | *Implementation Stage* | *Debriefing Stage* |

Program Activity*

- Apply for planning grant
- Identify generic goals common to individuals and groups involved
- Initial team-building

→

- Planning period
- Goals made specific with strong sense of common purpose
- Facilitator selected with trial period (to determine match/compatibility)
- Build trust among members
- Formalize rules of membership and member roles
- Administrative assistant selected

→

- Intense learning period
- Members learn more about each other

→

- Period of continued learning and planning for action
- Period of action designed to achieve goals

→

- Discuss changes, successes, challenges in learning
- Continue, refine, and possibly expand activities
- Possibly revisit and redefine goals

Evaluation Activity**

- Determine evaluation goals
- Hire evaluator

→

- Members keep "diaries" of observations about process

→

- Assess learning process and changes in participants
- Assess changes in policy or structure

→

- Assess client services
- Assess learning process and changes in participants
- Assess changes in policy or structure

→

- Assess changes in client services
- Assess changes in client outcomes

Figure 8.6   Model for Ideal Learning Groups Process

SOURCE: Adapted from Kreuter, M., Lezin, N., & Young, L. (2000).

staff. Because the Colorado experience shows that professionals are willing to devote, without much funding, considerable time toward advancing their individual and collective learning, expanding this model would seem to be possible and desirable. There appear to be particular opportunities in communities where members of the learning groups have many advantages to gain from their interaction and when these professionals are not coming from settings where there already is communication overload.

Adapting this model to other community service arenas is most likely to be successful when the facilitators are well matched to the style and content needs of each learning group. Creating a common vision within each learning group is also a critical first step, one that should be fostered early in the program, preferably before funds are requested. Group members must also realize that participating in such a group will require that they defer their passion for direct client assistance to spend time away from the day-to-day requirements of running a home visitation program.

Finally, to maximize the community-wide benefits of the learning groups model, the first phases of the learning period should focus on service delivery improvements and opportunities for changing client outcomes as well as on incorporating process and outcome evaluation methods. All of these processes will ultimately be enhanced when the period of learning is adequately funded to reflect the full program costs.

References

Chinman, M. J., Anderson, C. M., & Imm, P. S. (1996). The perceptions of costs and benefits of high active versus low active groups in community coalitions at different stages in coalition development. *Journal of Community Psychology, 24,* 263–274.

Gray, B. (1991). *Collaborating: Finding common ground for multiparty problems.* San Francisco: Jossey-Bass.

Korfmacher, J., O'Brien, R., Hiatt, S., & Olds, D. (1999). Differences in program implementation between nurses and paraprofessionals providing home visits during pregnancy and infancy: A randomized trial. *American Journal of Public Health, 89,* 1847–1851.

Kreuter, M., Lezin, N., & Young, L. (2000). Evaluating community-based collaborative mechanisms: Implications for practitioners. *Health Promotion Practice, 1,* 47–61.

Kumpfer, K., Turner, C., Hopkins, R., & Librett, J. (1993). Leadership and team effectiveness in community conditions for the prevention of alcohol and other drug abuse. *Health Education Research, 20,* 359–374.

Olds, D., Eckenrode, J., Henderson, C., Jr., Kitzman, H., Powers, J., Cole, R., Sidora, K., Morris, P., Pettitt, L. M., & Luckey, D. (1997). Long term effects of home visitation on maternal life course and child abuse and neglect: Fifteen year follow-up of a randomized trial. *Journal of the American Medical Association, 278,* 637–643.

Olds, D., & Hill, P. (1998). *Six-month progress report on Colorado Trust Grant Number 97048, Home Visitation Program Development in Colorado and Dissemination of the Home Visitation 2000 Study Findings.* Denver: University of Colorado Health Sciences Center.

9

What Do the Case Studies Say About Community-Based Health Promotion?

Douglas V. Easterling

Kaia M. Gallagher

Dora G. Lodwick

As defined in Chapter 1, *community-based health promotion* is a philosophy that emphasizes the role of community residents and community-based organizations in developing and implementing strategies to promote local health. The seven case studies described in the preceding chapters provided a fuller and more complex picture of the practical reality of community-based health promotion.

One of the most striking findings from the case studies is the diversity of approaches that local organizations can adopt to improve the health of their communities. In some of the initiatives, the funded agencies sought to improve health-related behaviors by implementing traditional public health interventions such as awareness raising, screening, health education, and prenatal counseling. In other initiatives, the grantees implemented a broader array of interventions targeted toward outcomes as varied as parenting, social support, self-esteem, and allowing seniors to remain in their homes. In addition, some of the initiatives employed a collaborative process of problem solving in which community stakeholders played an explicit role in making key project decisions.

The wide variation in approaches observed across the seven case studies might suggest to some readers that "community-based health promotion" is an amorphous or even ill-defined concept. In this chapter, we distinguish between a number of distinct (and sometimes competing) conceptualizations of what it means for a project to be "community based." Rather than adopting any single perspective, we argue that community-based health promotion is actually a multidimensional construct, involving issues such as the venue for the intervention, the type of organization that develops and implements the intervention, and the role of local residents. It is possible for a health initiative to be community based on some dimensions but not others. Moreover, as an initiative becomes more community based, there is a tendency for the intervention to address a broader scope of issues and to include more multidimensional strategies.

This chapter also discusses the challenges that community-based health promotion raises for evaluation. Community-based health initiatives typically adopt comprehensive strategies that address entrenched behaviors, lifestyle choices, economic conditions, and/or social structures. By their nature, these initiatives entail long time horizons and rely on the coordinated action of multiple stakeholders operating in different segments of the community. Because the action plans tend to be complex and ambitious, there is no guarantee of achieving success. *Documenting* success is arguably an even more elusive task.

At the end of this chapter, we address options for evaluating the effectiveness of a community-based health initiative from both a short- and long-term perspective. Based on the results from the book's seven case studies, we suggest that measuring changes in *community capacity* provides a useful approach for assessing whether or not a community-based initiative is on the path toward improved community health. This concept of "capacity" is illustrated by reviewing some of the key findings from the seven case studies.

Whereas the current chapter examines what we have learned about the concept of community-based health promotion, the final chapter of the book presents a set of practical recommendations for improving the practice of health promotion at the community level.

Dimensions Underlying Community-Based Health Promotion

In considering the approaches to health promotion adopted within the seven different initiatives, it might appear that each is premised on a somewhat different interpretation of the concept of "community-based health promotion." Some initiatives can be categorized as community based because health was promoted in a community setting rather than in a more medically oriented clinical setting. Others fit under the rubric of community based because organizations other than health departments or large institutions assumed a leadership role in developing and managing the interventions. Still others can be considered community based because local residents were given responsibility for making major decisions regarding the intervention. In other words, "community based" might refer to either (a) the venue of the intervention, (b) the type of organization carrying out the intervention, or (c) the role of community residents. In what follows, we describe how the three elements of community-based health promotion are manifested through the seven initiatives described in the previous chapters.

VENUE FOR INTERVENTION

Almost without exception, the initiatives described in our case examples were undertaken by grantees who conducted their health promotion activity in "community" settings rather than in more traditional health care environments. For example, the community-based organizations and local health departments funded under the Community Action for Health Promotion Initiative (CAHPI) (Chapter 5) operated within "the community," conducting activities such as conferences, workshops, health fairs, blood pressure screenings, and exercise classes. Likewise, some of the CAHPI grantees relied on the public airwaves or print media to raise awareness around specific health issues.

Other chapters provided additional examples of how health can be promoted in nonclinical settings. In the Colorado School Health Education Initiative (CSHEI) (Chapter 7), school districts adopted health education curricula, such as "Know Your Body," that provide basic instruction in health concepts to elementary school students.

In the Colorado Healthy Communities Initiative (CHCI) (Chapter 2), one community developed a program by which the health department maintained a diabetes education module on computers located in the local public library.

In the Teen Pregnancy Prevention Initiative (TPPI) (Chapter 4), many of the grantees operated within free-standing organizations and provided case management services and referrals to other service arenas for pregnant and parenting teens.

In a few instances, the health promotion initiatives described were carried out in neighborhoods and home environments. For example, the service providers who participated in Home Visitation Learning Groups (HVLG) (Chapter 8) visited young mothers in their homes to provide education and counseling on issues such as infant health and parenting. Likewise, agencies funded under the Volunteers for Rural Seniors Initiative (VRSI) (Chapter 6) delivered services such as home maintenance and meals on wheels to seniors within their homes.

LEAD ORGANIZATION

As noted in the introductory chapter, the term "community based" connotes much more than *where* health promotion activities occur. A community-based approach to health promotion also implies that actors other than health-related institutions have been given a critical role in the design and implementation of the overall project.

In funding these seven initiatives, The Colorado Trust sought to increase the number and diversity of organizations that would assume responsibility for designing and implementing health promotion activities. In initiatives such as CSHEI, the recipients of the grant funds were school districts. The HVLG project convened representatives of social service agencies that provide home visitation services within their communities. In initiatives such as VRSI, and CAHPI, eligibility for funding was more open-ended, leading to a broader cross section of grantees that included government agencies, nonprofit organizations, churches, and neighborhood associations. Some of these grantees were overtly oriented toward the cause of "health" (e.g., the county health departments funded under CAHPI), whereas others regarded health as only one component within a more comprehensive mission.

Collaboration offered another avenue by which non-health organizations became involved in the design and management of health promotion activities. The Colorado Trust required extensive community-wide collaboration among grantees funded under CHCI and TPPI. As such, these two initiatives, as well as the Community Indicators Project (Chapter 3), vested representative community coalitions with the authority to determine how health would be promoted within their individual community settings. To the extent that these coalitions afforded an authentic voice and decision-making role to community representatives and smaller, more grassroots organizations, health promotion could be considered to be even more community based.

ROLE OF LOCAL RESIDENTS

The third dimension of community-based health promotion involves a consideration of *who* at the local level has been empowered to make critical decisions and to design and carry out the program. Baker (1997) argues that the term "community based" should be reserved for those initiatives that are "primarily driven at every stage by the residents of the community." Although many public health interventions strive for "authentic" participation on the part of the community residents whose interests are being served, few efforts have actually achieved this objective (Baker, 1999; Novick, Brownson, & Baker, 1999). Particularly when health departments, universities, and other large institutions initiate the health promotion process, local residents are often relegated to an "advisory" role. In terms of Arnstein's (1969) "ladder of citizen participation," local residents rarely move past the rung of "placation" to a level where they are truly empowered to decide which health issues will be addressed and which interventions will be adopted.

The principle of citizen participation was a cornerstone for at least some of the initiatives described in this book. CHCI provides the clearest instance of local residents being organized to plan, design, and implement health promotion activities, with the principle of civic participation being central to this initiative. The first step in the CHCI process was to recruit a broad cross section of local citizens to become full and equal members of the stakeholder group that would be responsible for developing the action plan. In practice, some stakeholders were found to be more influential than others. Indeed, some residents dropped out of the process because the planning model process was perceived as being too elaborate or analytic. By and large, however, the action plans that emerged from the CHCI planning processes were developed by local residents who were working to promote the quality of life of the entire community.

In TPPI, The Colorado Trust required that residents representing all points of view in the community be included as stakeholders in the local TPPI collaboratives. To varying extents, this objective was achieved within the different TPPI projects. Although many of the stakeholders represented organizations such as the local health department, social service agencies, schools, and churches, there was also involvement on the part of community residents and parents of teens, especially during the planning phase of the 5-year project. Young people were engaged in a more sporadic fashion.

A similar pattern was found for CSHEI, where parents, along with teachers, participated on health education advisory committees. Community members were observed to be more likely to participate in the process of selecting curricula in communities where the topic of health education generated controversy.

In CIP, the funding agency emphasized the importance of selecting a set of indicators that would appeal to the values and priorities of the entire community. To achieve this objective, some CIP grantees included residents on their advisory committees. However, because of the technical nature of the indicator selection task, the members who remained engaged in the process tended to be those individuals with expertise in either research methods, comprehensive planning, or a content area such as economic development, natural resources, or human services. To reach a broader cross section of the community, some projects held forums to inform local residents about the concept of community indicators and to ask for recommendations. In all cases, the CIP projects disseminated reports summarizing the indicator data to residents (through media, forums, presentations to community groups, etc.) with the expectation that they would use the data to carry out (or at least support) actions to improve the health and quality of life of the community.

The three remaining initiatives (VRSI, HVLG, and CAHPI) were more deliberately focused on improving health promotion within the context of existing community organizations than they were on stimulating citizen participation. As such, the primary actors and decision makers in these initiatives tended to be agency professionals. VRSI involved citizens as volunteers in carrying out the programs but not in the planning and design of strategies. HVLG exclusively involved service providers who were brought together to determine ways in which their services could better serve their respective communities.

Likewise, most of the grantees in CAHPI were local health departments and established nonprofit organizations. At the same time, however, the managing agency (Colorado Action for Healthy People) also sought to identify fledgling grassroots organizations that could be mobilized to undertake health promotion projects. The best illustration of this strategy occurred in the rural town of Wray, where a group of parents came together to address the problem of drinking and driving among local teens. With the help of the managing agency, the parents recruited residents from throughout the community to support their efforts to convert a local storefront into a teen center.

Clarifying the Concept of Community-Based Health Promotion

Chapter 1 presented "community-based health promotion" as a shift away from more medically oriented techniques and paradigms, a shift that also expands the role of community residents. Each of the seven initiatives described in this book fits within this philosophy. As summarized in the previous sections, we believe that there are three dimensions regarding how community-based health promotion interventions are structured that uniquely define this philosophical approach:

- A shift in the venue of the intervention (from clinical settings to community settings)
- A shift in the type of organization that takes the lead in developing and implementing the intervention (from health-related institutions to community-based organizations)
- A shift in the locus of decision making (from experts to community residents)

Table 9.1   The Paradigmatic Shifts Associated With Community-Based Health Promotion

	From:	*To:*	*And Ultimately:*
Venue for intervention	Clinical settings (e.g., physician's office, health clinic, hospital)	Workplace School Non-health organizations Public forums Media (e.g., television, newspaper, billboards)	Neighborhood Home
Organization responsible for developing strategy	State health department Local health department Health care organization	Nonprofit organization Social service agency School district Coalition of agencies	Neighborhood association Church, synagogue, etc. Community development corporation Informal grassroots group
Role of local residents	Residents are simply clients for an expert-defined intervention	Residents are consulted by professionals in the development of the program	Residents control the process through which the program is developed and operated

Table 9.1 shows these paradigmatic shifts in more detail.

At a minimum, community-based health promotion is simply a shift away from the more traditional operationalization of public health in ways that provide more opportunities for the community's voice to enter into the design and management of programs. In its more advanced forms, community-based health promotion involves a group of residents taking their own initiative to make critical decisions about how to improve their own health, with these decisions leading to interventions that are subsequently carried out by community-based organizations within neighborhood settings.

These three dimensions tend to be interrelated in practice, but they refer to conceptually distinct aspects of the health promotion process. As such, it is possible for a health promotion initiative to be "community based" along one dimension but not another. For example, consider the case where a local health department designs and manages an infant mortality reduction program in which peer counselors go door-to-door in a low-income neighborhood. This program would be community based in the sense of operating within the community (i.e., the venue for health promotion) but not necessarily so when taking into account who designed the intervention.

The notion of "community based" can become even more complex when considering the perspective of players that operate outside the community. For example, funders often regard an initiative to be community based if the grantee has been given the prerogative to make the key strategic and programmatic decisions. In other words, "community based" is simply a contrast to "funder defined." Likewise, university researchers often use the term "community based" to refer to projects that take place off campus. Within this perspective, the "community" is everything that exists beyond the walls of the institution. As such, a project is community based if the major decisions are made by *external* organizations or individuals—even if the organizations involved are health related and/or the key decision makers are experts on the topic. It is easy to construct examples where an initiative would be community based from this perspective but not in terms of the role of local residents.

We point out these distinctions in definition because they explain the confusion that often surrounds health initiatives that take place in community settings. To an increasing degree, groups representing the interests of neighborhoods, communities of color, individuals with disabilities, and the poor have become active in calling for public health to become more community based (Baker, 1999). This perspective calls for those individuals whose health is at risk to be directly involved in the decision-making process. On the other hand, the term "community based" often has a weaker meaning among the other actors involved in designing and carrying out public health initiatives: local, state, and national health agencies; health care organizations; private foundations; and university-based researchers. Some of the individuals working from these perspectives regard an initiative to be community based if the intervention is carried out in a community setting. Others recognize the importance of citizen involvement but consider it sufficient to institute a process where a few residents "advise" the local health department on critical health decisions. These weaker definitions of "community based" will inevitably clash with the expectations and aspirations of those who advocate for a greater citizen role in project decision making.

Community-Based Initiatives
Expand the Health Promotion Paradigm

The previous sections of this chapter suggested that "community based" is not an all-or-nothing concept. Some health projects are community based only in the sense that the interventions are placed in community settings, whereas others reflect significant input (and even control) on the part of community residents. Moreover, this variation in the level of "community basedness" appears to have major implications for the type of health promotion strategies adopted by a community. Namely, as program planning and decision making become more decentralized and inclusive, the interventions chosen to be implemented tend to adhere less and less to traditional public health models.

For example, most of the local health departments funded under CAHPI developed programs focused on fairly traditional risk factors such as smoking, lack of exercise, and poor nutrition. Although the interventions were placed in community settings, most were developed by program managers within the grantee agencies and resembled the types of health promotion programs implemented by health departments across the country. In contrast, many of the community coalitions in CHCI and TPPI adopted a much broader perspective on the question of how health problems might be addressed.

In this section, we consider two distinct patterns that emerged in these initiatives, namely, that (a) the health promotion interventions developed by non-health organizations tended to address factors that went well beyond the standard health risk factors and (b) planning groups that were more broadly representative of the larger community tended to embrace a more holistic definition of health than typically emerges from the biomedical paradigm.

INTERVENING ON NONMEDICAL LEVERAGE POINTS

Not surprisingly, when non-health organizations begin to address health issues, they tend to adopt non-health strategies. In those initiatives designed to involve a broad range of community-based organizations (as opposed to simply recruiting health agencies), the resultant programs went beyond trying to change health behavior and individual risk factors. Many of these grantees sought to influence health by addressing cognitive, emotional, social, environmental, and even socioeconomic factors.

In VRSI, the funded agencies provided a host of supportive services (e.g., yard work, house cleaning, home maintenance, companionship, "meals on wheels," adult day care) that addressed the senior clients' physical environment or increased the clients' sense of social support. Rather than treating specific health conditions, these programs promoted health by helping seniors to maintain their independence to allow them to continue to live in their homes.

To address issues such as violence and childhood injury, some of the non-profit organizations funded under CAHPI employed strategies such as mentoring, counseling, and youth centers. The rationale underlying these programs was that providing at-risk youth with more social support, more encouragement for academic success, and more opportunities for constructive use of their time would reduce their impetus to engage in risky activities such as carrying a gun, drinking alcohol, using illegal drugs, and driving while intoxicated.

The TPPI coalitions also developed strategies that promoted "life options" for teens at risk for becoming pregnant. Several communities, for example, developed teen centers and recreation programs available to a broad spectrum of teens within their communities. In addition, a statewide public awareness campaign was initiated that stressed the importance of open, frank communication between parents and their teenage children regarding sexuality. These prevention-oriented interventions were designed to address the psychological, social, and economic risk factors associated with teen pregnancy. It is particularly noteworthy that the TPPI project directors from the five funded sites collectively incorporated the Search Institute's "developmental assets" philosophy into their programming. Under this approach, health promotion is viewed as only one aspect of a larger community-building effort:

> Ultimately, rebuilding and strengthening the developmental infrastructure in a community is not a program run by a few professionals (though they are certainly part of the team). It is a movement that creates a community-wide sense of common purpose, placing community members and leaders on the same team moving in the same direction. In the process, it creates a culture in which all residents are expected and empowered to promote the positive development of youth. (Benson, 1995, p. 11)

Thus, whereas a traditional health program might focus on modifying a specific set of behaviors that have been linked to narrowly defined health outcomes, grantees with broader missions tended to address a wider range of issues within a broader array of settings, often working to achieve change that would benefit a larger, more diverse segment of the community.

RECONCEPTUALIZING "HEALTH"

The case studies presented in this book suggest that health promotion takes on an even more global and comprehensive scope when the strategies emerge from the deliberations of a representative group of community stakeholders. In two of the chapters, those describing CHCI (Chapter 2) and TPPI (Chapter 4), citizen-based stakeholder groups were given the primary responsibility for designing the health promotion interventions that would receive funding. In discussing the factors that contribute to health, these groups brought up issues such as poverty, racism, lack of jobs, crime, environmental quality, and the social pressures associated with population growth and community conflict.

This broader health promotion agenda was particularly apparent in CHCI. As originally formulated, the CHCI model explicitly embraced the World Health Organization's broad definition of "health," where physical health is regarded as only one dimension among many that leads to a "healthy community." Moreover, the model views these dimensions as being strongly interrelated: Communities with healthy populations are assumed to also be strong in terms of economics, environmental quality, civic participation, and arts and culture. As a result, the CHCI stakeholder groups were encouraged to consider a broad array of factors and forces related to their communities' quality of life.

CHCI also called for an inclusive approach to decision making that respected the voices of all participants, regardless of their level of formal expertise or credentials. This principle of inclusivity was reinforced by the professional facilitators who helped the stakeholder groups to develop their action plans.

For all of these reasons, the grantees in CHCI developed strategies that addressed "whole system" factors rather than focusing solely on improving physical health. Indeed, as the example in the text box illustrates, some of the CHCI projects might seem to be only tangentially related to health.

Promoting Health Through Mass Transit

The Healthy Mountain Communities (HMC) project covers the resort region extending from Aspen down the Roaring Fork Valley to Glenwood Springs and then down the Colorado River to Parachute. The primary issue for this project, during both the planning and implementation phases, has been the region's rapid population growth. To manage growth-related problems such as traffic congestion, poor air quality, unaffordable housing, and loss of wildlife habitat, HMC convened regional forums on transportation and land use. Through this work, new state enabling legislation was passed allowing the formation of a regional transportation authority that supports the second largest bus system in the state (Larson, Christian, Olson, Hicks, & Sweeney, 2002).

Although mass transit certainly falls beyond the purview of traditional health promotion, this strategy might be the highest leverage approach to addressing air pollution. Similarly, a number of other CHCI projects determined that they could not promote health in isolation of the social, economic, and environmental conditions that influence the life of a community.

Community indicators provided another mechanism for CHCI grantees to address community problems according to a "systems" perspective. In CIP, grantees were encouraged to identify a diverse set of indicators that would measure the community's health and well-being. Drawing on the data sets maintained by many different agencies, the indicators projects created "big picture" reports that demonstrated the interrelationships among factors such as infant mortality, poverty, violence, unemployment, land use, cancer rates, and air quality. The intent here was to stimulate more coordinated, comprehensive problem solving on the part of elected officials, community organizations, and residents.

SUMMARY

These examples suggest that as community organizations and residents become more directly engaged in developing and implementing health promotion strategies, the analysis and deliberations become quite expansive:

- Organizations and residents that are not wedded to the medical model tend to consider a broad range of social, psychological, economic, and political factors when identifying the pathways to improved health. These include both *internal* factors (e.g., knowledge of community resources, self-esteem, sense of belonging) and *contextual* factors (e.g., prosocial school environment, supportive families, connected neighborhoods, inclusive civic infrastructure) that make it easier for individuals to achieve health.
- Planning processes involving a wide variety of stakeholders often produce a long and diverse list of factors that contribute to health.
- With laypersons involved in the decision-making process, "health" is often defined in broad terms (akin to "quality of life") as opposed to focusing on reductions in morbidity and mortality.

For all of these reasons, community-based health initiatives tend to produce complex interventions. Rather than focusing on health-specific knowledge, attitudes, and behavior, these interventions often aim to generate broad-based improvements in the conditions that face local residents. Correspondingly, the initiatives operate simultaneously on multiple leverage points at various levels (e.g., individual, school, neighborhood, community).

In sum, community-based health promotion portends a stretching of many of the conceptual and practical boundaries that demarcate the field of public health. When churches, schools, nonprofits, and neighborhood groups play a substantive role in health promotion, a very wide range of individual change and community change strategies come into consideration. Traditional public health activities such as immunization clinics, restaurant inspections, health fairs, mobile screening vans, brochures, and media campaigns continue to have a role in promoting community health. However, when health promotion is "community based" in the strongest sense of the term, the new players will invariably call into question many established principles regarding what "health" is and how it is created. Taken to the extreme, community-based health promotion may look more like *community development* than it does *public health*.

Evaluating the Success of Community-Based Health Initiatives

As noted previously, community-based health initiatives tend to generate complex, wide-ranging interventions that presume a long-term change process. Although a comprehensive holistic approach might be necessary to develop effective interventions (Stokols, 1992), this broadening in scope also complicates the evaluation process (Connell, Kubisch, Schorr, & Weiss, 1995; McKinlay, 1996). The evaluators of community-based health initiatives face considerable challenges in documenting health improvements, certainly when compared with researchers who are engaged in clinical trials or even quasi-experimental studies of model programs. In this section, we describe some of these difficulties and argue for the use of "proximal" indicators of success—shorter term outcomes that occur on the way to more tangible improvements in health status. We look specifically at *community capacity* as a proximal measure in evaluations of community-based health initiatives and then summarize how capacity was increased in the seven initiatives presented in this book.

THE EVALUATION DILEMMA

Perhaps the greatest obstacle to evaluating the outcomes of community-based initiatives is the time lag between programmatic activities and improvements in health status. For example, many of the initiatives described in this book began with a planning step during which community residents or program managers came together to understand their communities' issues in more depth and to develop what they believed would be effective and appropriate strategies. In instances where representativeness and inclusivity were emphasized, it often took a year or longer before programs were actually implemented.

Even with an efficient planning process, the programs developed under a community-based approach often have long time frames for achieving changes in health status. For example, the public awareness campaigns of some of the TPPI-funded communities were designed to foster more open communication between parents and youth around issues of sexuality. The logic was that with this increased communication, teens would be better informed when it came time to make decisions about sex and contraception. Assuming that this intervention had a positive effect on the knowledge, attitudes, and behavior of adolescents, one would not expect to see changes in community-wide fertility rates until years later.

A similar dilemma occurred in CSHEI. The health education curricula selected by the local health advisory committees were designed to instill a set of beliefs and attitudes in elementary school students that would reduce risk behaviors during adolescence and adulthood. Even if those interventions are effective, positive health outcomes might not emerge for many years. Moreover, even if those outcomes do occur, an evaluation might not be able to detect the change due to all of the competing influences on adolescent health that obscure the impact of health education delivered during children's earlier years.

It is even more difficult to document positive health outcomes when the intervention attempts to alter the overarching community context within which residents live their lives and experience health (Connell et al., 1995; Goodman, Wandersman, Chinman, Imm, & Morrissey, 1996; McKinlay, 1996). For example, most of the CHCI projects attempted to introduce a community forum or some other mechanism that would increase citizen participation in local affairs. Although the stakeholder groups anticipated that this type of work would improve local health, concrete outcome data will undoubtedly be slow to emerge. Furthermore, even if community health does improve, it will be difficult to isolate the contribution of the CHCI projects in producing this change.

PROXIMAL INDICATORS OF "SUCCESS"

There is no simple solution to the problem of detecting the "success" of community-based health initiatives. So long as community-based organizations and local residents develop ambitious interventions that operate in complex social systems, evaluation will be an imprecise endeavor. Nonetheless, it is possible to take steps that will improve the prospects of obtaining concrete answers to the question, "How well is the initiative working?"

One of the most useful strategies for focusing the evaluation of community-based initiatives is to specify the underlying "theory of change" that links the health promotion activities to tangible health outcomes (Weiss, 1995). With this approach, the designers of the intervention clarify the intended "change process" and create a map that traces the pathways through which the desired changes are expected to occur. By charting out the change process, this map will also suggest a set of mile markers. These mile markers represent the early effects of the initiative—outcomes that occur more immediately in response to the intervention and are instrumental in producing the health improvements that are the ultimate aim for the intervention. In identifying the key mile markers, one is providing the evaluation with a set of *proximal measures* of success.

For example, in the health education programming described previously, it was assumed that if students learn about the health consequences of factors such as diet, exercise, smoking, and substance abuse, they will be more willing to adopt healthy behaviors. In and of themselves, increases in knowledge are unlikely to be sufficient to guarantee behavioral effects, but they can be regarded as a necessary first step. Thus, improved knowledge is an initial mile marker on the path to long-term healthy behavior. By evaluating whether or not change occurs at this level, one is able to provide an initial sense of the intervention's effectiveness. Over time, evaluations can test for change along other indicators that are more directly connected to the ultimate desired outcome (e.g., attitudes and behaviors that are associated with less use of tobacco or alcohol during the middle school years).

Proximal Indicators at the Initiative Level

So far, we have been considering proximal indicators in the context of single-site evaluations. Proximal indicators are also useful in evaluating community-based initiatives at a more macro level. In particular, consider the perspective of the funder of the seven initiatives described in this book. The Colorado Trust was motivated first and foremost by a desire to improve the health of the communities where the initiatives were implemented. However, for all the reasons cited previously, the initiative evaluations were generally unable to show that these intended improvements in health status had actually occurred by the end of the initiatives. Rather, the evaluations focused on the shorter term, more direct effects of the initiatives—effects that set the stage for longer term health improvements.

Each initiative had its own predefined indicators of success (both short term and long term) based on the respective theory of change guiding the initiative. For example, in VRSI, success was gauged in the short run by testing for an increase in the use of volunteers among the funded agencies. The evaluation showed that some (but not all) of the grantees improved their systems for managing volunteers, recruited more volunteers, and used their volunteers to provide additional services to seniors in the community.

Although each initiative was evaluated according to a different set of proximal indicators, there were some commonalties across the seven initiatives. At the most fundamental level, all seven initiatives were designed to improve the *number* and/or the *effectiveness* of health promotion activities occurring within the funded communities.

In some initiatives, the funder was interested in expanding the use of specific health promotion strategies. For example, CSHEI was intended to increase the number of Colorado school children who received health education in the classroom. The initiative succeeded in stimulating 21 school districts to adopt health education curricula, although only a fraction of the teachers in those districts actually taught the full curricula to their students.

In other initiatives, the funder had more open-ended expectations with regard to increasing the number of health promotion activities carried out in the funded communities. In CAHPI, grantees were supported in implementing various strategies for addressing specified health issues such as violence, tobacco use, nutrition, and heart disease. Likewise, TPPI led to major increases in programming aimed at reducing adolescent fertility rates and improving birth outcomes among teen parents. And CHCI generated an average of six new health-related activities in each of 27 different communities (with "health" broadly defined).

The communities participating in these initiatives implemented not only more health promotion activities but generally more carefully planned and executed activities than would have occurred in the absence of the initiatives. This was particularly true of the initiatives that required grantees to undergo a planning process (e.g., CHCI, TPPI, CSHEI). By design, programs and strategies were selected and funded only if they appeared promising to a wide cross section of local stakeholders. Thus, one of the major benefits of these initiatives was not so much that *more* health programs were added but rather that communities introduced new strategies that appeared to be relevant to local conditions and likely to prove effective in promoting the health of the communities. In other words, the *addition of promising health promotion activities* served as an important early marker of "success."

In two of the initiatives, the focus was not so much on adding new health promotion activities as it was on *improving existing programs and services.* As mentioned earlier, VRSI supported community organizations in enhancing their programs through the increased recruitment and retention of volunteers. The HVLG initiative provided more intensive technical assistance to promote program improvement. By involving program managers in a structured multi-session exploration of the assumptions, strengths, and weaknesses underlying their home visitation services, this initiative led to significant changes in design and implementation as well as to the adoption of new evaluation strategies. As such, HVLG succeeded in terms of the *improved programs* indicator, which serves as the initial step on the path to improved health outcomes among clients in the community.

Community Capacity as a Proximal Indicator

So far, we have focused on the degree to which the seven initiatives described in this book achieved progress in terms of more health promotion programs and more effective programs. However, as indicated in Chapter 1, these initiatives were designed to affect not only *programs* but also the *capacity* of communities to address their own health issues. Whereas program-related outcomes are specific to the task at hand, capacity-related outcomes pertain to the community's ability to develop and carry out health strategies over the long run. Increasing community capacity may represent an even more significant contribution on the part of a funder than do improvements in individual programs (Goodman et al., 1998).

Assuming that community capacity is a critical indicator of success, the question arises as to what this concept actually refers to. Different analysts have chosen to operationalize community capacity in different ways (Parker, Eng, Schulz, & Israel, 1999). The Aspen Institute (1996), for example, refers to a framework of "commitment, resources, and skills" that are hypothesized to facilitate community problem solving. Likewise, Goodman et al. (1998) conceive of capacity as "assets to address the presenting health concerns."

As noted in Chapter 1, The Colorado Trust employed a definition that referred to "the set of assets or strengths that residents individually and collectively bring to the cause of improving local quality of life" (Easterling, Gallagher, Drisko, & Johnson, 1998, p. 7). Consistent with the Goodman et al. (1998) taxonomy, the foundation's conceptualization of community capacity focused on the following five specific dimensions:

1. Skills and knowledge that allow for more effective actions and programs

2. Leadership that allows a community to draw together and take advantage of the various talents and skills that are present among its residents

3. A sense of efficacy and confidence that encourages residents to step forward and take the sorts of actions that will enhance the community's well-being

4. Trusting relationships among residents that promote collective problem-solving and reciprocal caregiving ("social capital")

5. A culture of learning that allows residents to feel comfortable in exploring new ideas and learning from their experience

These dimensions of capacity can conceivably be developed at many different levels in any given community: among a select set of individuals, within a funded organization, within a community coalition, or across the larger community.

CAPACITY BUILDING ACROSS THE SEVEN INITIATIVES

In general, the evaluation studies included in this book found that the seven initiatives did lead to increased *capacity*—at the individual, organizational, and community levels. For example, the evaluation of CAHPI found that the funded agencies increased their capacity to design and implement health promotion projects, particularly in the areas of program administration, collaborating with other agencies, and promoting their programs through the media. Likewise, through repeated stakeholder meetings and periodic community forums, the stakeholders involved in TPPI established closer working relationships and established a greater sense of common purpose. And in CHCI, the survey of stakeholders documented increased capacity among local residents in the areas of planning, analysis, and collaborative problem solving.

Table 9.2 provides a summary of how community capacity was built across the seven initiatives. The left-hand column of the table lists the five dimensions of community capacity (knowledge and skills, leadership, collective efficacy, social capital, and culture of openness and learning) and provides more specific descriptions of what it would mean to build capacity according to each dimension. For example, *leadership* would increase either if new leaders emerged from within the community or if existing leaders developed stronger leadership skills. The remaining seven columns in the table show which forms of capacity were built within each of the initiatives. An uppercase bolded "X" indicates that the evaluation provides "strong" evidence that at least some of the funded communities increased the respective form of capacity through their involvement in the initiative. A lowercase unbolded "x" indicates that the evaluation provides "limited" evidence that some communities experienced an increase in capacity. It should be noted that the ratings in this table are subject to the limitations of each initiative's respective evaluation design; some evaluations may have failed to detect particular increases in capacity simply because these dimensions were not explicitly related to one of the funder's evaluation questions.

The first and fourth rows of Table 9.2 suggest that at least some forms of community capacity are nearly guaranteed to increase over the course of a community-based health initiative. Namely, simply as a result of being involved in a grant-funded project, program managers experience an increase in their knowledge, skills, and leadership. Community-based projects breed growth and learning, particularly for managers who are new to the work. This effect was demonstrated explicitly in the CAHPI evaluation, which found that the least experienced program managers scored the greatest gains in skill levels.

Networking between sites (which was incorporated into all seven of the initiatives) enhanced this skills development process. To the extent that the initiative provided intensive technical assistance to the grantees (e.g., CSHEI, HVLG), there was even stronger growth in knowledge and skills among project staff (including those who came into the initiative with years of experience).

None of the other forms of community capacity increased as consistently as did program managers' skills, knowledge, and leadership. This is not surprising given that program managers are the individuals who are most connected to, and thus most affected by, an initiative. Once we move out beyond

Table 9.2   Increases in Capacity Across the Seven Initiatives

	CHCI	CIP	TPPI	CAHPI	VRSI	CSHEI	HVLG
Knowledge and skills							
1. The program managers and service providers in the funded agencies increased their managerial skills, particularly in the areas of program planning, grant writing, evaluation, public education, and advocacy.	X	X	X	X	X	X	X
2. Coalition members developed new planning and problem-solving skills.	X	X	X			x	
3. Community residents became more aware of local issues.	X	X	X	x	x	x	
Leadership							
4. Project staff developed stronger leadership skills, especially with regard to facilitative leadership.	X	x	X	x	x	X	X
5. New leaders emerged from within the community.	X	x	X	x	x	x	x
Collective efficacy							
6. In communities that had traditionally relied largely on well-established institutions, residents and community-based organizations took the initiative to institute strategies or programs to meet their needs.	X	x	X	x		x	
Social capital							
7. Stronger, more trusting relationships were formed among community residents, particularly across sectors or population groups.	X		X			X	
8. Stronger, more trusting relationships were formed among service providers, leading to more collaborative behavior and better coordination of services.	x	x	X	x	x	X	X

(Continued)

213

Table 9.2 Continued

	CHCI	CIP	TPPI	CAHPI	VRSI	CSHEI	HVLG
Culture of openness and learning							
9. Community residents were exposed to (and listened to) the perspectives of people they do not normally interact with.	X		X		x	x	
10. Organizations developed new data systems to evaluate the effectiveness of their programs.		x	X	x	x	X	X
11. Communities instituted measurement systems to monitor quality of life.		X	X				

NOTE: CHCI = Colorado Healthy Communities Initiative; CIP = Community Indicators Project; TPPI = Teen Pregnancy Prevention 2000 Initiative; CAHPI = Community Action for Health Promotion Initiative; VRSI = Volunteers for Rural Seniors Initiative; CSHEI = Colorado School Health Education Initiative; HVLG = Home Visitation Learning Groups initiative. An uppercase bolded "**X**" in the cell indicates that there is strong evidence that the respective initiative built this form of capacity in at least some funded communities. A lowercase unbolded "x" in the cell indicates that there is limited evidence that this form of capacity was built in at least some funded communities. A blank cell indicates that it is unlikely that this form of capacity was built through the initiative.

214

the immediate project staff (e.g., collaborating organizations, stakeholders in the planning process, the community at large), the effects became less consistent across initiatives. Most of the initiatives achieved at least some increase in capacity at these larger levels, such as a new evaluation system within the funded organization, increased community awareness around health issues, and the emergence of new leaders. However, only two of the initiatives, CHCI and TPPI, made major inroads in building the capacity of the larger community. Not surprisingly, these were the initiatives with the most inclusive strategic planning processes. The two other initiatives where residents were somewhat less involved in a strategic planning process, CIP and CSHEI, showed somewhat less of an effect with regard to community-level awareness, leadership, relationships, and/or learning.

The between-initiative differences in capacity building are consistent with the different theories of change that define the initiatives. CAHPI and VRSI were aimed at promoting new and/or improved health programs among individual organizations. Thus, it is not surprising that the observed increases in capacity relate primarily to changes in those organizations and their staff.

At the other extreme, CHCI, CIP, TPPI, and CSHEI were designed to advance *community problem solving* at the same time that new health promotion strategies were being introduced into settings such as schools, family resource centers, public agencies, nonprofit organizations, and neighborhoods. By bringing together diverse stakeholders to develop consensus-based strategies, these initiatives were able to achieve outcomes such as increased social capital and collective efficacy, at least among the participants in the process.

The final initiative, the HVLG project, was a hybrid of these two general models. The HVLG initiative brought together program managers from multiple agencies to improve their respective programs.[1] Correspondingly, most of the increased capacity accrued within individual organizations. However, the collaborative learning process also established the groundwork for ongoing coordination of services between agencies. In one instance, the process even facilitated the design of a comprehensive community-wide approach to serving the needs of families at risk for child abuse.

In an overall sense, the seven initiatives promoted capacity building at the individual, organizational, and community levels. In some initiatives, the effects were more narrowly focused on individual and organizational capacity at the grantee level: health-specific knowledge, program development skills, leadership, strategic thinking, volunteer recruitment, board development, and evaluation systems. In other initiatives, the effects extended out to the larger community: expanded awareness and knowledge on the part of residents regarding local issues, increased social capital, greater community consensus, and "community will" with regard to improving health conditions. However, in all cases, there was at least some evidence that the initiatives provided the funded communities with an increased ability to identify and address their most pressing health issues.

THE SIGNIFICANCE OF INCREASED COMMUNITY CAPACITY

Given that the seven initiatives increased the capacity of the participating communities, the question arises as to whether this is a meaningful outcome with respect to improved health status. An increase in community capacity will lead to improved health through at least three theoretical pathways. First, if communities develop more leadership and collective efficacy, they will be more likely to take the initiative in developing health promotion strategies. Second, if community members increase their skills, knowledge, and opportunities for learning, they will develop health promotion strategies that are more likely to be effective in improving health status. Third, if social capital increases, local residents will find themselves in a more supportive, caring environment, which in turn will reduce stress and improve their ability to cope with illness.

A growing body of empirical research demonstrates the validity of these pathways. In particular, communities that have higher levels of "capacity" (as defined here) tend to have better levels of health (Easterling et al., 1998). For example, in a study of U.S. cities, LaVeist (1992) found that "political empowerment" within the African American community had a positive influence on child health (e.g., lower levels of neonatal mortality). Likewise, a study of violence in Chicago found that rates of violence varied across neighborhoods as a function of "collective efficacy," defined as the willingness of residents to intervene in instances of threat or criminal behavior (Sampson, Raudenbush, & Earls, 1997). In addition, there is strong correlational evidence that social capital influences health status. Namely, in the United States, those states where residents report more trusting relationships and more civic participation tend to show lower levels of mortality, both in an overall sense (i.e., age-adjusted mortality rates) and for specific causes of death (e.g., infant mortality, heart disease, malignant neoplasms) (Kawachi, Kennedy, Lochner, & Prothrow-Stith, 1997).

Studies such as these suggest that if communities experience a significant increase in their capacity (e.g., social capital, collective efficacy), they will eventually see improvements in their physical health status.[2] As such, social capital and other forms of community capacity can serve as proximal indicators to evaluate whether a community-based health initiative is on the road to improving the health of the community (Kreuter, Young, & Lezin, 1998; Lomas, 1998; Petersen, 2002). Particularly given the long time horizon that characterizes the community-based approach to health promotion, funders may need to be satisfied with increased community capacity as evidence that their initiatives are "working."[3]

Although increased capacity can be viewed as an important step toward improved community health, this effect by itself is not sufficient to produce significant changes in health status. Capacity provides the groundwork for developing health promotion strategies that are appropriate for local conditions, priorities, and values. However, for those strategies to be effective, they need to be designed intelligently, implemented in a rigorous manner, and sustained over time. In the final chapter of this book, we present concrete and practical guidance for achieving these outcomes and, more generally, for increasing the effectiveness of community-based health promotion.

Notes

1. One of the HVLG grants went to a single organization, the Mesa County Health Department, which used the learning process to improve and reconcile the home visitation services provided by the various nurses in the department.

2. If we adopt the broader definition of "health" adopted by the World Health Organization (1995), which includes social, political, economic, and environmental dimensions in addition to physical and mental health, it is even more likely that increased levels of capacity will pay off in the form of improved health. In particular, Putnam (2000) presents an extensive body of literature documenting the relationship that social capital (defined in terms of trusting relationships and civic participation) has on nearly every facet of a community's quality of life.

3. Funders that are narrowly focused on the mission of improving physical health might find it necessary to demonstrate more than simply an increase in community capacity. Namely, a community that increases its capacity to solve problems might devote its attention to issues other than health, disregarding the intent of the funder that financed the capacity-building process.

References

Arnstein, S. R. (1969, July). A ladder of citizen participation. *Journal of the American Institute of Planners, 54,* 216–224.

Aspen Institute. (1996). *Measuring community capacity building: A workbook in progress for rural communities.* Washington, DC: Author.

Baker, Q. E. (1997). *What does community based mean?* (briefing paper). Durham, NC: Center for the Advancement of Community Based Public Health.

Baker, Q. E. (1999, Summer). Understanding the community in CBPH. *Voices From the Field,* pp. 1–2. (Durham, NC: Center for the Advancement of Community Based Public Health)

Benson, P. L. (1995). *Uniting communities for youth.* Minneapolis, MN: Search Institute.

Connell, J. P., Kubisch, A. C., Schorr, L. B., & Weiss, C. H. (Eds.). (1995). *New approaches to evaluating community initiatives: Concepts, methods, and contexts.* Washington, DC: Aspen Institute.

Easterling, D., Gallagher, K., Drisko, J., & Johnson, T. (1998). *Promoting health by building community capacity: Evidence and implications for grantmakers.* Denver: The Colorado Trust.

Goodman, R. M., Speers, M. A., McLeroy, K. A., Fawcett, S., Kegler, M., Parker, E., Smith, S. R., Sterling, T. D., & Wallerstein, N. (1998). Identifying and defining the dimensions of community capacity to provide a basis for measurement. *Health Education and Behavior, 25,* 258–278.

Goodman, R., Wandersman, A., Chinman, M., Imm, P., & Morrissey, E. (1996). An ecological assessment of community-based interventions for prevention. *American Journal of Community Psychology, 24,* 33–61.

Kawachi, I., Kennedy, B. P., Lochner, K., & Prothrow-Stith, D. (1997). Social capital, income inequality, and mortality. *American Journal of Public Health, 87,* 1491–1498.

Kreuter, M. W., Young, L. A., & Lezin, N. A. (1998). *Measuring social capital in small communities.* Atlanta, GA: Health 2000.

Larson, C., Christian, A., Olson, L., Hicks, D., & Sweeney, C. (2002). *Colorado Healthy Communities Initiative: Ten years later.* Denver: The Colorado Trust.

LaVeist, T. (1992). The political empowerment and health status of African-Americans: Making a new territory. *American Journal of Sociology, 116,* 364–375.

Lomas, J. (1998). Social capital and health: Implications for public health and epidemiology. *Social Science Medicine, 47,* 1181–1188.

McKinlay, J. B. (1996). More appropriate evaluation methods for community-level health interventions. *Evaluation Review, 20,* 237–243.

Novick, L. F., Brownson, R. C., & Baker, E. A. (Eds.). (1999). *Community-based prevention: Programs that work.* Gaithersburg, MD: Aspen Publishers.

Parker, E. A., Eng, E., Schulz, A. J., & Israel, B. A. (1999, Fall). Evaluating community-based health programs that seek to increase community capacity. *New Directions for Evaluation, 83,* 37–54.

Petersen, D. (2002). The potential of social capital measures in the evaluation of community-based health initiatives. *American Journal of Evaluation, 23,* 55–64.

Putnam, R. (2000). *Bowling alone: The collapse and revival of American community.* New York: Simon & Schuster.

Sampson, R. J., Raudenbush, S. W., & Earls, F. (1997). Neighborhoods and violent crime: A multi-level study of collective efficacy. *Science, 277,* 918–924.

Stokols, D. (1992). Establishing and maintaining healthy environments: Towards a social ecology of health promotion. *American Psychologist, 47,* 6–22.

Weiss, C. H. (1995). Nothing as practical as good theory: Exploring theory-based evaluation for comprehensive community initiatives for children and families. In J. P. Connell, A. C. Kubisch, L. B. Schorr, & C. H. Weiss (Eds.), *New approaches to evaluating community initiatives: Concepts, methods, and contexts* (pp. 65–92). Washington, DC: Aspen Institute.

World Health Organization. (1995). *WHO Healthy Cities: A programme framework.* Geneva: Author.

10

Practical Lessons for Promoting Health at the Community Level

Douglas V. Easterling

Kaia M. Gallagher

Dora G. Lodwick

The evaluation findings presented in Chapters 2 through 8 demonstrate that communities funded under the seven community-based health promotion initiatives took important steps to address local health issues. These results add to the body of evidence supporting the value of community-based health promotion. However, the evaluation studies also found that communities face formidable challenges in developing and implementing health promotion strategies that are both locally relevant and effective in achieving their objectives. Building on the lessons and implications presented at the end of each case study chapter, this final chapter presents a set of overarching recommendations for advancing the practice of community-based health promotion.

Our recommendations are organized around a set of five challenges that frequently arise in initiatives where communities strive to develop solutions to their health issues. Two of these challenges pertain to individuals and organizations working within the communities (e.g., local health departments, non-profit organizations, neighborhood groups, elected officials, individual residents): (a) *inclusiveness of the process* and (b) *effectiveness of the strategy.*

Two other challenges pertain to the funders that support the health promotion work of communities (e.g., state and federal health agencies, grantmaking foundations): (c) *controllability* and (d) *adding value*. The fifth challenge relates to the interaction between community groups and funders. Namely, given the fact that funders and grantees often bring two different sets of interests, expectations, and notions of "accountability" to their relationship, they may find it difficult to create strong *partnerships* with one another.

These five challenges are described in more detail in the following sections. For each challenge, we draw on the seven case studies to provide examples of how the core issues might be addressed.

In focusing on these five challenges, our recommendations are intended to complement and add to the substantial body of literature that already exists on the topic of improving health promotion at the community level (e.g., Bracht, 1990, Connell, Kubisch, Schorr, & Weiss, 1995; Fawcett et al., 1995; Fetterman, Kaftarian, & Wandersman, 1996; Gorin & Arnold, 1998; Green & Kreuter, 1990; Hawkins & Catalano, 1992; Kreuter, Lezin, Kreuter, & Green, 1998; Linney & Wandersman, 1991; Minkler, 1997). These texts provide theoretical frameworks and practical advice for addressing the major challenges that arise in developing and carrying out health promotion programs, such as finding effective interventions, implementing program models with fidelity, recruiting participants, recruiting and managing staff, sustaining programs at the end of grant funding, evaluating how well programs are meeting their expectations, and improving programs based on evaluation findings. A 1999 report issued by Grantmakers in Health provides corresponding advice for organizations that fund health promotion programs (Praeger, 1999). This publication identifies a number of "elements of success" that health funders should strive to achieve, including a coherent sense of purpose, in-depth knowledge of the field, a clear theory of change, strategic deployment of resources, and mobilization of communities.[1]

The recommendations that we have derived from the seven community-based initiatives funded by The Colorado Trust are largely consistent with the advice offered by these earlier publications. However, we believe that the evaluation studies included in this book provide additional insights that can improve the practices of community groups and funders. As more communities and funders experiment with the community-based approach, we expect that the recommendations presented here will be enhanced even further.

Challenges and Lessons for Communities

The community-based approach to health promotion is premised on the principle that persons living within a community should be involved in deciding which health issues are most crucial to address and how those issues should be addressed. This emphasis on local control is intended to increase the likelihood that health promotion strategies will be relevant and appropriate to the local context. At the same time, however, developing health-promotion strategies within a community-based context also brings a set of challenges, two of which are discussed in this section:

1. Achieving broad, active community participation in the design and implementation of health promotion programs

2. Developing maximally effective health promotion strategies

ENSURING AUTHENTIC PARTICIPATION ON THE PART OF THE LARGER COMMUNITY

The hallmark of community-based health promotion is active and authentic involvement on the part of those persons whose health is at stake. In the initiatives described in this book, a variety of community stakeholders were engaged in the planning and implementation of health programs, including adolescents, parents, teachers, neighborhood associations, business owners, representatives of specific ethnic populations, and community residents. According to the philosophy underlying community-based health promotion, widespread community involvement increases the chances of developing a strategy that will (a) be relevant to the priorities of the community, (b) reach the intended individuals, (c) deliver an appropriate message, and (d) achieve the desired response.

Barriers to Participation

Although public participation is a desired component in many community-based health initiatives, local residents are rarely the most active or influential participants in designing and carrying out programs. Typically, an initiative to promote a community's health is managed by a local health department or some other health-related agency or nonprofit organization, with most key decisions being made by the board and staff of this organization.

Even when health organizations make a "good faith" effort to involve local residents, participation is often modest or intermittent. Given the competing demands from work, family, children's schools, and other religious and civic organizations, many residents are unable to set aside time to become involved in something as complex and time-consuming as a community health initiative.

Although it is easy to attribute low public involvement to a lack of personal interest, it is also important to consider the barriers that are created (often unwittingly) by organizations that seek citizen participation. In particular, health-related planning processes, and community coalitions more generally, can suffer from the following shortcomings:

- Meetings are scheduled at times that are inconvenient for residents (particularly those with children or highly structured jobs).
- Meetings are held in agency environments that are uncomfortable or intimidating to nonprofessionals.
- Deliberations and decision making are conducted with an emphasis on technical expertise, prior experience, and analytic logic, effectively ignoring the perspective of citizen representatives.

In short, when local residents participate in coalitions or collaboratives, they may find themselves adapting to a foreign culture that is at odds with their more familiar ways of thinking and interacting. This clash of cultures can become further compounded when there are differences in race, ethnicity, and socioeconomic status among the participants (Kreuter & Lezin, 1998). Moreover, if the community has been characterized by a history of racial discrimination or disenfranchisement, an institutionally driven health promotion initiative may be viewed with mistrust among some segments of the community. Thus, barriers to participation can stem not only from the specific project at hand but also from the larger social-political context that defines how people perceive and respond to one another.

Strategies for Increasing Community Participation

The initiatives presented in this book, particularly those that included stakeholder groups or community advisory committees, provide some useful lessons for addressing these challenges of inclusion and participation. These lessons go beyond the more obvious remedies such as public education and outreach by responding directly to the barriers that are most likely to discourage broad-based community participation.

Relevant Health Issue. For local residents to become involved in a health-promotion project, they must first feel some commitment or urgency regarding the purpose of the project. In other words, community participation presupposes that the health issue being addressed is relevant to the community. This is less likely to occur in projects that are driven primarily by the availability of grant funds. Local agencies and nonprofit organizations sometimes pursue funding opportunities without assessing the larger community's willingness or readiness to devote attention and resources to the designated health topic. If a grant is awarded under these conditions, the recipient organization may find it quite difficult to involve any more than a narrow segment of the community in the project.

To ensure broad-based community participation, assessments of public sentiment should be conducted prior to committing to a particular health issue. Such an assessment might be carried out through door-to-door surveys of neighborhood residents or by meeting with the membership of neighborhood associations, churches, or civic organizations.[2] Alternatively, a local agency might begin with an open-ended planning process where a broad cross section of residents are invited to help determine the community's health priorities.

Inviting Participation Early in the Process. The most direct means of ensuring that community members have a strong stake in a health project is to involve them at the very early stages. In some projects, public representatives are invited in *after* the planning group has resolved critical issues such as the health issue that will be addressed, the nature of the problem-solving approach, the players who will be involved, the timing of the decisions, and even some of the elements of the strategy. Some individuals might be satisfied in simply being part of a well-defined project, but many others are apt to stay away because they are under the impression that this is someone else's idea. A broader level of commitment and "buy-in" on the part of local residents requires that they be brought into the process at an early stage when the procedures for planning and problem solving are still being established.

Authentic Role for All Participants. Given the substantial time commitment required by most community health projects, it is important that the participants believe that their involvement is contributing to the development and/or implementation of the strategy. Whether participants are elected officials, health professionals, or concerned residents, their roles in shaping and/or carrying out the initiative need to be substantive and meaningful. At a bare minimum, this means that all participants must have some degree of decision-making responsibility and authority. To the extent that residents are equitably represented in leadership positions, it will be easier to ensure that the initiative respects the voices and viewpoints of the community at large.

Flexibility and Respect for Differences. Even if individuals are granted an authentic role in a project's decision-making processes, they might feel alienated by the way in which the project is carried out. Full participation on the part of community residents is more likely to be achieved when consideration is given to the timing and setting for meetings, the manner in which those meetings are conducted, and the language that is used to talk about issues. These meeting logistics and arrangements should be designed so that they are conducive to community representatives' ways of thinking and interacting while also accommodating their fundamental needs with respect to work schedules, child care, and transportation.

Community residents often have needs and expectations that are quite different from those of the professionals who are accustomed to planning and implementing health projects. Whereas an agency manager might be accustomed to a tightly run meeting in a conference room, residents might be much more comfortable with more open-ended discussions in a church basement or someone's living room. Sharing a meal may be regarded as a critical part of bringing people together within certain neighborhoods but might not even be a consideration for other members of the planning group.

Cross-cultural differences can come into play with regard to a whole host of issues that arise in designing and carrying out a community health initiative. These might include the protocol for discussing an issue, the rules for decision making, and the use of technical information such as health surveillance data. Open discussions should be held at the outset to identify the expectations of the different group members and to find ways in which to accommodate each person's most important interests. The ultimate goal of these efforts, irrespective of how they are carried out, is to ensure that no one with a stake in the initiative feels excluded from participating because the process has been set up in an uninviting or even intimidating manner. This requires a deliberate effort to understand the varying needs and worldviews of the different participants.

DEVELOPING EFFECTIVE
HEALTH PROMOTION STRATEGIES

By definition, a community-based health promotion effort acknowledges and incorporates the views of community members whose health is at stake. "Outsiders" with expertise in the topic of the initiative may also be involved, but their role is primarily to support the planning and decision making of stakeholders from the community. The presumption here is that local actors have direct knowledge of the conditions and opportunities facing their community and, thus, are in the best position to identify the community's most important health issues and to develop effective solutions.

In this section, we consider the validity of this proposition. Namely, does the community typically come up with the best possible solution to its health issues? Although there is some evidence that community-based interventions are not always effective in achieving positive health outcomes (Oetting & Beauvais, 1991), the seven case studies in this book provide many examples of communities taking effective action. In our view, the critical question is not whether the community-based approach is effective in any absolute sense but rather under what conditions community groups produce effective health promotion strategies.

In this section, we present four recommendations for improving the ability of community groups to develop and carry out effective health promotion strategies:

1. Conduct a strategic analysis of the health issue prior to deciding on the solution.

2. Tap into both scientific knowledge and community knowledge to identify potentially effective strategies.

3. Map out and test the logic of possible programs to decide which one(s) is most likely to succeed in achieving the desired health outcomes within the local context.

4. Evaluate how well the programs work in practice, reflect on the findings, and improve the health promotion strategy on an ongoing basis.

By incorporating these recommendations, the community-based health promotion model becomes grounded within a broader base of knowledge about effective program interventions and, thus, becomes capable of producing the outcomes that communities are hoping to achieve.

Conducting a Strategic Analysis

Strategic analysis is essentially a process of answering pointed questions. These questions probe the community group's understanding of the health issue at hand and how positive change can occur with respect to this issue. There is no standard set of guiding questions that will serve the interests of every organization or coalition, but the following questions may be useful in a variety of situations:

- In simple and concrete terms, what is the health issue to be addressed?
- Which measures provide a valid picture of how the community has been affected by this health issue?
- Where in the community is this health issue most evident?
- What factors are associated with making the problem worse in some areas?
- What factors seem to protect against the problem?
- What trends (e.g., social, demographic, economic, political) influence this health issue—for either the better or the worse?
- What needs to change in the community to address this issue?
- More specifically, how can change occur? Toward which groups should change efforts be directed?
- What opportunities for achieving those changes already exist within the community?
- What types of intervention are likely to promote the desired changes?
- How feasible is it to achieve those changes given (a) the financial resources and scope of influence available to those involved in the change effort, (b) the possibility of partnering with additional individuals and organizations concerned with this issue, and (c) the social, political, and economic climates of the community?

This type of investigatory process is designed to yield a health promotion strategy that focuses on the most critical *strategic leverage points* (Senge, 1990) and relies on programs and activities that are capable of influencing those leverage points.

In the public health model, strategic leverage points are often equated with *risk factors*, defined as conditions that increase the likelihood that a particular disease or illness will occur in an individual or a population. In identifying a strategic leverage point, one looks for a risk factor that (a) has a powerful effect on the health condition of interest and (b) can be influenced by the persons and organizations involved in the project, given their resources, knowledge, and position (Green & Kreuter, 1990). For example, many of the home visitation programs represented in the Home Visitation Learning Groups (HVLG) initiative were designed to reduce the incidence of child abuse by addressing risk factors such as poor parenting skills and a lack of social support.

Leverage points can be more than simply *negative* conditions to be remedied (e.g., poor eating habits, lack of knowledge, lack of willpower, economic deprivation). Health can also be promoted by taking advantage of key opportunities that are present in the community such as an integrated network of health care clinics, a strong community-wide ethic of physical fitness, and a shared sense of responsibility for the well-being of all residents. The Volunteers for Rural Seniors Initiative (VRSI) (Chapter 6) was designed explicitly around the positive leverage point of *untapped volunteers* as a means of improving the health and well-being of seniors living at home. Leverage points might also include the "protective factors" identified by Hawkins and Catalano (1992) or the "developmental assets" promoted by the Search Institute (Benson, 1997): individual characteristics, social supports, and environmental conditions that allow youth to resist the pressure to engage in unhealthy behaviors such as substance abuse, violence, and promiscuous sex.

Identifying the most critical strategic leverage points requires an in-depth understanding of both the health issue being addressed and the community context. To develop such an understanding, one might carry out steps such as quantitative and qualitative assessments of local conditions, a review of the relevant health promotion literature, strategic thinking exercises, and extensive deliberation. Carrying out these activities provides a "picture" of the various factors that contribute to the health issue, which in turn can help the sponsoring organization or coalition to determine where it should intervene to have the greatest impact on the topic of concern.[3]

Two of the initiatives, the Colorado Healthy Communities Initiative (CHCI) (Chapter 2) and the Teen Pregnancy Prevention 2000 Initiative (TPPI) (Chapter 4), engaged local stakeholders in a planning process that explicitly sought out strategic leverage points. After exploring their local health issues through community assessments and in-depth deliberations, the stakeholder groups identified a relatively small set of factors on which to focus their health promotion activities ("key performance areas" in the case of CHCI, "strategic goals" in the case of TPPI). In addition, the Community Indicators Project (CIP) (Chapter 3) encouraged each participating community to identify the interrelationships among the different aspects of quality of life and then to channel local resources toward those factors that would provide the greatest leverage in improving overall quality of life.

Strategic analysis is a critical first step in defining the objectives and parameters of the health promotion programs that will be carried out. Although this might seem like an obvious recommendation, it is not always followed. Program models are adopted for a variety of reasons such as familiarity, expediency, and the influence of key stakeholders. For a program to be effective in achieving improvements in community health, it needs to operate on those leverage points that are most relevant for that community. Once leverage points have been identified, local planning groups are in a position to determine which program models are most appropriate.

Using Both Scientific and Community Knowledge to Develop Effective Strategies

In selecting or designing a health promotion program, one of the fundamental questions is, "Which strategies will achieve the greatest impact on the critical leverage points (i.e., those that contribute most to the health issue) given the context of this particular community?" Although it is possible that the community might need to develop a completely new approach that fits the local context, a review of existing programs often brings an appropriate strategy to the surface. This review should include the following steps:

1. Compile a list of programs that other communities have adopted to address the health issue.

2. Look for programs that address the strategic factors that the group has focused on.

3. Consider the available research evidence for those programs.

4. Determine whether programs that appear promising based on prior experience are appropriate for the community.

5. Assess the community's ability to implement programs that appear to be promising and appropriate.

According to Morrissey et al. (1997), many community groups fail to conduct an adequate review of existing programs (especially the evaluation data associated with those programs) prior to arriving at their own program decisions:

> A significant limitation to program success has been the quality of programs delivered to the community. Program practitioners have not consistently used information regarding the science of effective prevention programs in the selection and implementation of interventions. (p. 368)

It should be acknowledged, however, that conducting such a review can be time-consuming, particularly for practitioners and community residents who are not well versed in the relevant research literature. These types of searches are more manageable when researchers have already compiled an independent review. For example, the University of Colorado's Center for the Study and Prevention of Violence searched the literature for effective gun-prevention programs and then summarized the available evaluation data in a report designed to support community-based programming (Arredondo et al., 1999).

Learning how various programs have fared in other communities is a useful step toward developing an effective strategy. However, replicating "proven" program models might not be sufficient. Even if an evaluation study has shown that a program produces significant effects, that program might not be appropriate to the demographics, culture, or politics of a particular community. Moreover, many of the programs that have been shown to be effective require the staff to have a specific education background or specialized training (e.g., Olds et al., 1997). It may be difficult to find individuals with these credentials in small, rural communities.

In considering whether or not to adopt a particular health promotion program, planning groups should consider not only the available research evidence but also the question of whether or not a potential program would fit within the local context (Wandersman et al., 1998). This two-step process acknowledges that there is a place not only for scientific knowledge but also for the knowledge that community members can add regarding local conditions. As an example, the Colorado School Health Education Initiative (CSHEI) (Chapter 7) included a planning process that explicitly drew on both scientific and community knowledge.[4] In this initiative, each school district had a health education advisory committee (HEAC) charged with reviewing and selecting health education curricula for elementary, middle, and high school students. As a first step, the managing agency in the initiative provided each HEAC with a synopsis of the research findings for a number of highly regarded curricula. If an HEAC indicated that it wanted to consider a curriculum outside of this set, the managing agency searched for available research and summarized the findings for the HEAC. In making its final selection, each HEAC considered not only the scientific research but also the degree to which the material and approach contained within each curriculum fit within the institutional context of the school system and the cultural-political context of the larger community.

Mapping Out the Logic of Programs

One of the most important steps in choosing or developing a health promotion program is to map out the pathway(s) through which the program is expected to achieve its objectives. This can be done in the form of either a "theory of change" (Weiss, 1995) or a "logic model" (W. K. Kellogg Foundation, 1998). In either case, the objective is to identify the shorter term and longer term effects of the program and then to determine how and why those effects are likely to occur.

In Chapter 9, we introduced the concept of "theory of change" as a tool for evaluation. By laying out the chain of events that leads to the ultimate outcomes of interest, an evaluation can define markers of success during the early stages of the program. This process is also useful during the planning stage because it allows the program designers to examine critically the assumptions that under-lie the programs they are considering. By explicitly mapping out what is required to achieve its objectives, the group may decide that its program is unlikely to succeed, impractical, or inappropriate for the local community. This could lead to either a revision in the approach (e.g., by adding more frequent or intensive services) or a search for alternative program models.

Developing a theory of change or a logic model is an in-depth process that involves exploration, clarification, analysis, and a willingness to change direc-tion. Among the seven initiatives described in this book, the HVLG project devoted the greatest attention to this line of work. With the help of facilitators, the managers of home visitation programs took a hard critical look at the ser-vices they were providing and the likelihood that those services would achieve outcomes such as reduced child abuse and improved parenting. As a result of this process, a number of participants refined their program models to take into account the available research and to incorporate suggestions from other members of the learning groups.

Evaluating,, Learning, and Evolving

Regardless of how much planning, investigation, and analysis goes into the development of a health promotion strategy, it will invariably be imperfect. No program achieves everything that its designers hope to achieve. The recipients of health education or counseling interventions do not always change their behavior as quickly or profoundly as the program model presumes. Unforeseen obstacles emerge, slowing the implementation of certain compo-nents of the program (e.g., follow-up counseling) or even preventing the program from getting off the ground.

For all of these reasons, community-based health initiatives need to include systems for evaluation and learning. Any such system should include an assessment of how the program is actually being carried out (e.g., what services and activities are actually being delivered, how they are being delivered, who is receiving them) as well as an assessment of how the recipients of those activities are responding. Evaluation data provide an empirical picture of the program's outcomes and accomplishments as well as insights into where the program is not meeting its expectations and how it can be strengthened (Patton, 1997; Posavac & Carey, 1997). The "theory of change" process recommended earlier can provide a great deal of guidance in developing appropriate and focused evaluation questions.

By now, most organizations that carry out health promotion are well aware of the rationale and potential benefits of program evaluation. Funders and professional evaluators have published a number of textbooks and guidebooks to demystify the topic and to provide practical guidance on how to design and implement evaluations (e.g., Linney & Wandersman, 1991; W. K. Kellogg Foundation, 1998). Still, many community-based organizations struggle with both the feasibility and the usefulness of program evaluation (Baker, Davis, Gallerani, Sanchez, & Viadro, 2000; Fine, Thayer, & Coghlan, 1998).

If evaluation is to be a meaningful exercise for community-based organizations, more emphasis needs to be placed on the process of learning as opposed to simply judging whether or not a program has been "successful." For community stakeholders to view evaluation as an opportunity for learning, the evaluation needs to focus on outcomes and processes that they regard as relevant and interesting. This is more likely to occur if these individuals are directly involved during the initial planning stages in determining which questions will guide the evaluation (Fetterman et al., 1996).

In all of the initiatives described in this book, the funder encouraged grantees to conduct evaluations that would answer their critical questions. Three of the initiatives (TPPI, CSHEI, and the HVLG program) actually provided grantees with dedicated resources to plan and carry out their evaluations. Different grantees embraced evaluation with varying levels of enthusiasm, but in general these community organizations appeared to regard evaluation as more of an opportunity than an obligation.

This process of evaluation, learning, and refinement maximizes the chances that promising programs will reach their potential. More generally, all four of the steps proposed here—finding strategic leverage points, relying on scientific and community knowledge to develop effective programs, mapping out program logic, and evaluating/learning—complement one another in strengthening community-based health promotion. We believe that by incorporating these steps into the planning, implementation, and refinement of their health promotion strategies, community groups are more likely to achieve significant improvements in the health issue they are committed to addressing.

Challenges and Lessons for Funders

By definition, community-based health promotion is primarily the work of local residents and organizations. At the same time, the seven case studies described in this book demonstrate that community-based efforts can benefit from support provided by grantmaking foundations and government agencies, many of which are based outside the community. From the funders' perspective, however, the community-based paradigm raises distinct challenges. In this section, we focus on two specific dilemmas for funders:

- *Sharing decision making with grantees.* When a funder supports community-based health promotion, it is by definition encouraging grantees to find their own solutions to their own health issues. This approach reduces a funder's ability to control how its money will be spent and compromises its ability to evaluate the effectiveness of its grant making.
- *Helping from outside the community.* Although the community-based model presupposes a nondirective approach on the part of outsiders, foundations and government funders can offer grantees a great deal of valuable expertise. This raises the dilemma of how an outside funder can be helpful to a local project while still ensuring that the project is community driven and locally owned.

The remainder of this section presents a set of recommendations to funders as to how they can address these two challenges and become contributing partners in community-based health promotion.

SHARING DECISION MAKING WITH GRANTEES

The community-based approach requires that funders allow local stakeholders to make at least some (if not most) of the major decisions regarding which health issues to address, where to intervene, and which activities to carry out. This sharing of decision-making authority can raise a number of concerns for a funder, including the following examples:

- Community groups might spend their grant dollars addressing health issues in which the funder has little interest.
- The grantee organization might choose not to focus its project on the funder's target population.
- Grant dollars might be spent on programs that the funder believes to be ineffective or even on programs that the funder is opposed to on philosophical or ideological grounds (e.g., providing contraception to teens).
- The funder might find it difficult to establish clear a priori criteria by which to hold grantees accountable.
- It may be difficult to evaluate individual grantees in a multisite initiative according to a common set of outcome measures.

More generally, allowing community-based groups to make the critical decisions regarding program direction complicates the issues of stewardship and fiduciary responsibility for a funder.

Without minimizing the importance of any of these issues, funders can take a number of steps to manage the uncertainty that is inherent in community-based health promotion. In the remainder of this section, we consider three specific techniques: (a) deliberately considering the funding organization's commitment to community-based health promotion, (b) making an informed deliberate decision about where to impose requirements and where to "let go," and (c) including in the evaluation design outcomes such as organizational learning and community capacity that allow for a fuller assessment of the return that might result from the funder's investment in an initiative.

Does the Funder Have an Authentic Commitment to the Community-Based Model?

Community-based health promotion requires a funder to show a great deal of faith in the ability of community groups to determine the direction of their programs. Before making such a commitment, the board and staff of the funding organization need to ask themselves whether they genuinely believe that community-based organizations, agencies, or coalitions are in the best position to establish the health priorities for their communities and to develop health promotion strategies. Do they believe that these groups will reach informed conclusions and implement effective programs? If a community group chooses a strategy that appears to be inappropriate or ineffective to the board and staff of the funding organization, would they be willing to fund the implementation of that strategy?

Although these questions might appear theoretical at the outset of an initiative, they often become fundamental in defining what the initiative actually looks like in practice. Hence, the board and staff of the funding organization should seek to clarify their beliefs on these issues prior to establishing any expectations with grantees. TPPI provides an excellent example of how a funder's commitment to local control can be explicitly tested. During the process of planning this initiative, The Colorado Trust engaged a consultant who interviewed each member of the board and staff regarding their preferences and values on the topic. Rather than asking for a general assessment of the importance of local control, the interviews presented a range of scenarios where affording local control might have potentially negative consequences. These scenarios included one where a local stakeholder group chose a program that was unproven through rigorous evaluation studies and one where the stakeholders chose a politically controversial strategy (e.g., abortion counseling). After discussing the results of these interviews, the board members agreed that they would be willing to fund the action plan submitted by a TPPI stakeholder group so long as all of the members of the group were willing to sign a statement indicating that they approved of the action plan. Thus, the values clarification exercise allowed the foundation to develop a more fully refined set of principles regarding local control, one that relied heavily on the notion of community-wide consensus and buy-in.

Funders are more apt to grant discretion to a community group when that group has undertaken a thoughtful, inclusive planning process. However, each funder reaches its own conclusions about how much decision-making authority to allow its grantees. In large measure, a funder's choice will hinge on its beliefs about the capacity of its grantees. In particular, does the funder believe that local organizations and residents have the inherent capability to focus on the "right" issues, to find the "right" strategies, and to implement appropriately the chosen programs? If the answer is no or even "not sure," it may be difficult for the funder to carry out an initiative that allows community groups to determine which strategies will be supported with grant funds.

As the board and staff of a funding organization clarify their beliefs and assumptions regarding community capacity, they should consider not only the skills and expertise that already exist in the community but also the possibility that those skills and expertise might develop over the course of the initiative, particularly with the funder's assistance. *Community capacity* refers not only to a community's current ability to carry out effective health promotion activities but also to its potential to do this work (Goodman et al., 1998). Viewing community capacity as *potential* (both realized and unrealized) has practical implications when it comes to evaluating the success of a community-based health initiative. A community-based initiative may "fail" in the sense that the projects funded under the initiative produce weak results but "succeed" in the sense that the funded communities, through their experience with the initiative, increase their *long-term* ability to plan, develop, and implement programs. Whether a funder deems such an initiative to be an overall failure or an overall success will depend largely on the funder's values and the time horizon over which success is being judged.

It is clear that the community-based health promotion model will appeal to some funders more than others. Those who value concepts such as community capacity, civic engagement, community mobilization, and learning will be naturally drawn to the model. In contrast, funders with pre-established expectations or short time frames are unlikely to adopt a grant-making paradigm in which communities engage in a lengthy process of learning, experimenting, and refining their programs.

Retaining Control Over
Decisions the Funder Considers Critical

Although local control is the defining feature of community-based health promotion, a funder need not adopt a completely "hands-off" policy. A funder can still specify its own objectives and place certain constraints on the allocation and expenditure of funds. The challenge is to design an initiative that allows the funder to meet its objectives while still allowing grantees authentic control over decision making. In other words, the funder needs to find an optimal balance between control and letting go.

It is instructive to consider the different ways in which this balance was struck in the seven initiatives presented in this book:

- In TPPI, funding was restricted to the issue of teen-pregnancy prevention, but within this issue, grantees could select whichever interventions they thought best served the interests of their local communities.
- In the Community Action for Health Promotion Initiative (CAHPI) (Chapter 5), groups applying for grant funds devised their own strategies to address selected health topics such as smoking and injury prevention.
- In VRSI, grants could be used only to expand the use of volunteers, but this could occur within many possible program strategies (e.g., respite, meals on wheels, home maintenance) directed at a variety of specific health issues, so long as the applicant could demonstrate that the funded services would assist seniors in staying in their homes.
- In CSHEI grantees were required to use their funding to support health education in local schools, but local HEACs decided which curriculum would be used within elementary schools as well as which risk factors would be addressed through the middle and high school curricula that were selected.
- In CHCI and CIP, the funder prescribed the planning process, but there were no constraints regarding the issues or strategies that would emerge from this process (although The Colorado Trust provided implementation funding only for strategies that either addressed the Healthy People 2000 objectives or continued the healthy communities process).
- In the HVLG initiative, funding was earmarked for a "learning group" process among practitioners of home visitation, but the funded groups were free to choose their own model for the learning process as well as the outcomes toward which they were striving.

From this pattern of funding, it is apparent that there are three major decisions over which a funder can choose whether or not to exercise control:

- The health issue that the grantee will address
- The program strategy that the grantee will employ to improve health
- The process of decision making, planning, or learning that the grantee will undergo to develop health promotion strategies

Funders are unlikely to vest grantees with the full responsibility for making all three of these decisions because this situation would be tantamount to giving grantees carte blanche to use grant funds in whichever way they see fit. Most funders would find such an arrangement quite challenging, particularly when it came to the question of how to hold grantees accountable.

By carefully mapping out its ultimate aims and its underlying assumptions, a funder can better determine which decisions to control and which to relinquish to grantees. From the authors' perspective, the critical question is, "which arrangement is most likely to leave the community with a set of health promotion activities that will effectively address the community's most critical health issues and will be sustained over the long run?"

Establishing Consistent and Reasonable Criteria for Evaluating "Success"

With community-based health promotion, it is inevitable that grantees will vary in the health promotion strategies they adopt. Some grantees may have particularly ambitious objectives, whereas others may strive for more modest outcomes. A funder's grant monitoring system could inadvertently penalize those grantees with higher and perhaps unachievable goals. This is particularly problematic if a grantee's future funding depends on how much "success" is achieved with the current grant. For the grant monitoring system to be fair to all grantees, it is important that grantees be held accountable to a consistent set of criteria.[5]

Consistency in measurement is also important from the standpoint of evaluation. For a funder to obtain an overall assessment of what was accomplished within a multisite initiative, the evaluation should measure the amount of progress that each funded community achieves with regard to the objectives of the initiative. Even though different sites may adopt quite different strategies, the evaluation needs to employ a common metric to aggregate across sites and produce a reliable summary measure of how much change occurs.

In terms of either grant monitoring or evaluation, the critical challenge is to identify measurable concepts that are (a) true to the objectives of the initiative and (b) relevant to the work that each funded community has carried out under the initiative. One concept that satisfies both of these criteria is the *soundness* of the health promotion strategy that the grantees develop under the initiative. From the perspective of either the funder or the grantee, it is important that grant dollars be directed toward strategies that are designed soundly enough (in terms of scientific validity and community fit) to have the potential of achieving their objectives. "Soundness" might be measured in terms of the logic of the program model or the degree to which the strategy addresses the strategic leverage points identified by the planning group (Goodman, Wandersman, Chinman, Imm, & Morrissey, 1996; Wholey, 1994).

A funder can evaluate the success of a community-based initiative by assessing not only the strategies that grantees develop over the course of the initiative but also the degree to which the funded organizations (as well as other individuals in the community) increase their ability to develop effective solutions to health problems. The analysis of community capacity presented in Chapter 9 provides a number of ideas for specific dimensions that might be assessed: enhanced program development and managerial skills within funded organizations and coalitions, the emergence of new leaders within the community, and the development of stronger interconnections among local organizations and residents. Depending on the objectives of the particular initiative and the funder's perspective on the role of community capacity in promoting health, outcomes such as these might serve as reasonable indicators of whether the initiative has been effective in supporting the process of community-based health promotion.

HELPING FROM OUTSIDE THE COMMUNITY

Foundations and government funders have historically played a critical role in supporting community-based health promotion. This support comes not only in the obvious form of funding for health promotion programs, but also through activities that add value to the work of their grantees. By providing technical assistance that is relevant and effective, funders can help grantees to develop better strategies in a more efficient manner. By creating opportunities for grantees to network with one another, funders can accelerate each organization's learning process. And simply by virtue of their position overseeing multiple grantees in the same initiative, funders can see patterns and learn lessons that advance the work that takes place at the community level. In the following subsections, we expound on these ideas and suggest a number of mechanisms (in addition to grants) through which funders can assist community-based organizations and coalitions in accomplishing more than they could on their own. These recommendations build on the techniques that The Colorado Trust incorporated into the seven initiatives described in earlier chapters.

With all these recommendations, we have tried to remain sensitive to the fact that funders are often located outside the communities they fund. As an outsider, a funder may not fully appreciate the social-political climate within which its grantees operate (Sievers & Layton, 2000), and thus might inadvertently develop technical assistance approaches or collaboration models that grantees find inappropriate or even counterproductive. The approaches described below are specifically designed to be flexible and responsive to local conditions, and thus to support communities in achieving their own purposes.

Initiate the Process of Community-Level Health Promotion

Perhaps the most important role that a funder plays in community-based health promotion is to encourage local organizations and residents to take the initiative to address issues that affect the community's health. The case studies in this book clearly showed that, through its initiatives, The Colorado Trust was able to mobilize a large number of organizations and individuals across the state to focus more explicitly on the task of promoting health. In some initiatives, the foundation elicited interest in a specific health topic (e.g., teen pregnancy, smoking, violence), whereas in other cases, communities were activated to address the broader health and well-being of the communities. To the extent that health issues are underappreciated or underaddressed within a community, funders can play a crucial role in focusing local actors on opportunities for improving their quality of life.

Foster More Deliberate and Comprehensive Program Planning

One of most effective ways for a funder to promote community-based health promotion is to provide local groups with the resources and the rationale to conduct systematic planning and problem solving. In theory, communities do not need help from funders to carry out the type of strategic analysis and program development that was described earlier in this chapter. In practice, however, there usually needs to be some imperative before individuals and organizations will devote time and effort to such an involved process. Typically, that imperative comes from a funder.

Five of the seven initiatives included in this book (TPPI, CHCI, CIP, CSHEI, and the HVLG project) required the funded communities to conduct some type of planning or program development process as part of their grant.[6] These planning efforts typically involved participants from multiple organizations and/or sectors coming together around a common purpose, sometimes for the first time.

Many of the initiatives described in this book provided grantees with a specific model for planning or decision making. Depending on the initiative, the planning group carried out activities such as community health assessment, an environmental scan, an analysis of strategic issues, a review of the research literature, and the development of an action plan. These processes were designed to encourage community members to be deliberate and analytic as they identified critical health issues and developed health promotion strategies. The planning models also introduced communities to concepts such as stakeholder analysis, consensus decision making, learning groups, the World Health Organization's definition of health, and community indicators.

Offer Appropriate Forms of Technical Assistance

Particularly if funders are interested in supporting the capacity-building process within funded communities, technical assistance can yield high returns. Technical assistance consultants can help funded communities to become more knowledgeable about the specific health issues that are being addressed and also can assist grantees in becoming more skilled in program planning, collaborative decision making, project management, evaluation, marketing, and many other issues that influence the success of a a community based project. When communities receive technical assistance that is appropriately matched to their needs and culture, they are able to develop more effective health promotion strategies and, thus, to make more prudent use of their project funds. From a funder's perspective, then, technical assistance serves as a means of increasing the returns on the grant dollars invested in communities.

Communities can benefit from technical assistance at every step in the process of developing, implementing, and refining health promotion strategies. Technical assistance providers are particularly useful during the early stages when a community is determining its priorities and considering possible strategies. In TPPI, CHCI, and the HVLG initiative, The Colorado Trust paid for professional facilitators who helped the planning groups to explore issues, interpret data, carry out respectful deliberations, reach conclusions, and make decisions. In contrast, the planning processes in CIP and CSHEI were facilitated by the staff of local organizations. Even here, however, the foundation supported the process by providing these local facilitators with technical assistance consultants who helped them to develop their skills in community outreach, group facilitation, conflict resolution, and strategic planning.

In addition to facilitating the planning process, technical assistance providers can help the planning group locate relevant research studies, translate the findings to the local context, and develop a sound program model. In all of the initiatives described in this book, The Colorado Trust provided grantees with some degree of technical assistance on the health issues they were addressing.[7] Once the health promotion strategies were developed, the technical assistance providers assisted in areas such as program implementation, evaluation, project management, organizational development, marketing, grant writing, and sustainability.

Regardless of the issue or skill that is being addressed, technical assistance needs to be substantive enough to serve the needs of the grantee. Half-day workshops on topics such as diabetes prevention, community mobilization, and program evaluation will at best provide an introduction to the topic. To build skills and improve health programming, a funder will need to adopt a more systematic approach to technical assistance that engages grantees a number of times over the course of the initiative.

In developing a technical assistance strategy, a funder should also recognize the developmental nature of the capacity-building process. Technical assistance may need to be frequent and intensive during the early stages of an initiative when the community participants are at the steep end of the learning curve. However, this might also be the stage where grantees are most reluctant to admit that they need assistance, so the funder may need to take the lead in offering technical assistance opportunities. As the funded organizations become more experienced and confident, they will be more willing to request technical assistance that meets their specific needs. As the projects continue to unfold, the grantees may even begin to request forms of technical assistance that were not foreseen at the outset of the initiative.

Given the diversity of issues and community contexts that arise in most community health initiatives, it is useful to tailor technical assistance to the individual circumstances of each grantee. Although a group training session can be an efficient means of delivering information (particularly basic introductory knowledge), communities may encounter challenges that can best be addressed by having technical assistance providers travel to their sites and offer advice related to their particular needs. Assuming that budgets for technical assistance allow for multiple visits to each site, the consultants can take on the role of *coach* in actively guiding the grantee organizations through the various stages of their projects while also providing support and encouragement when the inevitable disappointments arise.

The case studies described in this book illustrate the value of this more tailored approach to technical assistance. The individuals who provided technical assistance in CAHPI, VRSI, CSHEI, and the HVLG initiative all described their role in terms of coaching, encouraging, and facilitating the grantees' learning process. In general, this support was greatly appreciated by the staff of the funded organizations, particularly in cases where (a) the communities were experimenting with a new approach, (b) the project staff were new to the work, or (c) the projects were surrounded by controversy or politics.

Foster Grantee Networks

Technical assistance consultants play a critical role during the initial stages of program planning and skills development. As community-based projects proceed, however, the individuals carrying out those projects develop their own expertise. On key issues such as community conflict, client recruitment, cultural appropriateness, staff and volunteer burn-out, and project sustainability, the grantees themselves often become "hands-on" experts who learn what works in their respective community contexts.

Providing grantees with opportunities to share their lessons with one another is an important mechanism for accelerating the development of effective health promotion strategies. Across the seven initiatives in this book, supporting grantee networks proved to be one of the most valuable contributions made by the funding organization. The Colorado Trust paid for grantees to travel to periodic meetings where they could discuss their experiences with one another. Funding was also made available to bring in experts from around the country who could provide suggestions on how to address issues such as developing and sustaining effective projects, marketing, and working with diverse populations.

In CHCI, the grantees created a new nonprofit organization dedicated to cross-project networking and promoting the healthy communities movement across the state. In TPPI, the grantees came together as a collaborative to create a statewide media campaign promoting parental involvement in their children's sexuality education. To varying degrees, grantees within all of the initiatives described in this book pointed to their networks and networking meetings as helping them to increase their capacity to manage and sustain health promotion projects.

Joint Challenge for Communities and Funders

So far in this chapter, we have described two major challenges that community-based health promotion poses for communities (i.e., authentic participation and developing effective solutions) and two major challenges that it poses for funders (i.e., sharing decision-making authority and helping from outside the community). In this section, we raise one final challenge that pertains to both communities and funders: creating authentic dialogue between funders and community grantees.

Recognizing that funders and community-based stakeholders start from different points of view can help both parties to communicate more directly about their respective interests and concerns. Community groups (especially grassroots organizations) are typically focused on the immediate needs of local residents, whereas government funders and grantmaking foundations tend to be concerned with the health and well-being of multiple communities, often covering a large geographic area. In evaluating the success of a community-based health initiative, grantee organizations will generally be concerned with the degree to which specific health promotion activities have been carried out or whether clients have changed particular sets of behaviors. Funders are likely to be concerned not only with the individual success of each project, but also cross-site comparisons and the aggregate effect of their grantmaking.

In addition to these differences in perspective and expectation, funders and grantees occupy quite distinct positions with regard to power and authority. Funders have the authority to give and take away money. This creates an undeniable imbalance of power between funders and the groups they fund. With that imbalance, a grantee may feel as though it is acting merely as an agent for the funder, carrying out activities that the funder expects (or that the grantee thinks the funder expects), even if those activities are not directly related to the interests of the organization or the community. In the remainder of this section, we suggest a set of constructive steps that grantees and funders can take to create a more positive partnership that meets the fundamental needs of both parties.

CLARIFYING AND COMPARING EXPECTATIONS

When a funding agency gives a health promotion grant to a community organization, it is fair to assume that the two parties have overlapping interests with regard to improving community health. As indicated earlier, however, funders and grantees have contrasting roles and perspectives that may complicate their ability to come into a community health initiative with fully compatible interests and expectations. Tension or confusion might arise around issues such as constraints on how grants may be used, the role of the lead agency, the likelihood of subsequent funding, and the definition of a "successful" project.

To resolve potential points of dispute, the first step is for both funders and grantees to clarify their own expectations. A funder should spell out in its grant announcement or request for proposals the requirements that funded organizations must meet while also identifying the decisions and issues that are being left to the community to resolve. When a funder is ambiguous on the scope of decision-making authority that is vested with grantees, grantees sometimes try to accommodate the funder's presumed interests rather than making decisions that are in the best interests of the community.

Once an initiative is under way, the funder and the grantees should schedule in-person meetings where they can talk through their specific expectations, concerns, and questions. This might be done as part of site visits to funded communities as well as during networking meetings where all of the grantees can meet with the funder to develop a common understanding of what will occur under the initiative and the overall objectives that the initiative is designed to accomplish.

One of the most important steps in this process of reconciling expectations is to probe for areas of potential disagreement or confusion. Funders should recognize that this can be a somewhat awkward and unnatural process for grantees. Given the importance of staying in good graces with their funders, most community organizations find it risky to raise challenging or direct questions. Nonetheless, creating productive partnerships requires that these conversations between funders and grantees be honest and open and that both parties take risks and make the effort to understand the other's perspective. It is also important to remember that the goal of these conversations is not to bring the interests of funders and the interests of grantees *completely* into alignment with one another. Because they differ in their perspectives and to whom they hold themselves accountable, funders and grantees are very likely to focus on somewhat different outcomes when judging the success of their shared endeavors.

SEPARATE AND COOPERATIVE LEARNING

Program evaluation often creates the context where funders and grantees are most acutely aware of their contrasting expectations. The chapters in this book summarize evaluation studies commissioned by The Colorado Trust to address the foundation's evaluation questions. These studies examined questions related to collaboration, community-based problem solving, capacity building, and the design and implementation of effective health promotion programs. Over the course of the initiatives, the funded organizations raised different types of evaluation questions related to how well their specific programs were achieving their objectives. In response, The Colorado Trust supplemented the initiative-level evaluations (which focused on the macro perspective) with funding and technical support to allow grantees to design and carry out evaluations to address their own questions and issues. In HVLG, this support came in the form of facilitators who helped the learning group participants clarify their evaluation questions and develop measurement systems. In TPPI and CSHEI, the foundation provided grantees with the opportunity to apply for supplemental funding to hire their own evaluation staff or consultants.

This "dual-track" approach to evaluation (simultaneously conducting an initiative-level evaluation and supporting the program evaluation efforts of grantees) explicitly recognizes that the funder and the grantees have distinct learning objectives within the same initiative. At the same time, initiative-level evaluation and "local" evaluation need not be incompatible. In fact, these two different levels of evaluation complement one another in providing a fuller picture of how the initiative has unfolded. Pooling the evaluation findings enlarges and enriches the perspectives of both the funder and the grantees.

When a funder and grantees come together to learn from their evaluation studies, they are creating a unique opportunity for synergistic thinking. By combining the perspectives of the funder, the community organizations, and the evaluator in a common conversation, this process has the potential to yield significant advances in the practice of community-based health promotion.

Conclusion

The seven case studies included in this book demonstrate the substantial potential for community-based health promotion to address critical health issues. Through methods such as collaboration, community-wide strategic planning, citizen advisory committees, public forums, and community indicators, many of the projects funded under these initiatives made significant progress in mobilizing their communities to address the myriad factors that impinge on health.

An important by-product of this collaborative problem solving has been the lasting ability it created among local residents to relate to one another in new ways—more collaboratively, openly, and directly. More generally, nonprofit organizations, government agencies, program managers, and residents increased their capacity to design and manage health programs. New leaders emerged not only among the organizations that were funded under the initiatives but also within the larger community. Local residents increased their awareness of the issues confronting their communities and what might be done to achieve positive change on those issues. Stronger interpersonal and interorganizational relationships were built throughout the funded communities. Perhaps most important, communities increasingly came to recognize what they were capable of accomplishing in addressing their own health issues.

Although these increases in community capacity are important outcomes, they are only intermediate steps toward improvements in community health. For initiatives such as the ones described here to create measurable changes in health status, community-based projects will need to maintain their momentum and become even more effective and strategic. This evolutionary process requires ongoing support from a host of community stakeholders as well as from funders.

Grants from foundations and government agencies can support community-based health promotion in a number of important ways: strategic planning, program development, demonstration projects, and evaluation. In addition to financial support, funders can provide a number of other resources that promote project success: technical assistance, networking, encouragement, and the sharing of lessons learned. At the same time, constructively supporting the process of community-based health promotion depends as much on a funder's orientation and style as it does on the specific resources the funder provides to grantees. The community-based approach calls for funders to show faith in the capacity of the groups they fund, even when there is evidence of confusion, conflict, or missed opportunities. The most important contribution that funders can make with regard to community-based health promotion is to support and interact with grantees in a manner that allows communities to grow and learn as fully and efficiently as possible.

In sum, community-based health promotion offers significant promise as an approach for improving the health of communities, yet the pathways to success are neither direct nor immediate. Perhaps it is unrealistic to expect any approach to be clean and straightforward given the intractable and thorny health issues that community-based health projects often address (e.g., violence, teen pregnancy, racial and ethnic disparities in health status). Community-driven health promotion does not guarantee immediate remedies to these problems, but it does offer the possibility of authentic solutions that become deeply woven into the fabric of the community over the long run.

Notes

1. The Milbank Memorial Fund's (1999) report, *New Foundations in Health: Six Stories,* describes the process through which six health foundations created during the 1980s and 1990s developed their grant-making strategies. These case studies suggest a number of lessons for funders with regard to enhancing the health promotion activities of grantees.

2. The Community Action for Health Promotion Initiative offered funding and technical assistance to help community organizations assess local residents' health priorities (under the "Needs Assessment" track of the initiative). Only a small number of organizations took advantage of this opportunity.

3. Kennedy, Braga, and Piehl (2001) show how a community-based collaborative in Boston employed strategic analysis to develop strategies that proved effective in reducing gun violence. The Boston project served as a role model for the Strategic Approaches to Community Safety Initiative, which was funded by the U.S. Department of Justice and implemented in 10 communities around the country (Coleman, Holton, Olson, Robinson, & Morrison, 2001).

4. Another good example of this blending of science and community discernment occurred with The Colorado Trust's Colorado Violence Prevention Initiative. In this initiative (not included in the current book), technical assistance providers from the University of Colorado's Center for the Study and Prevention of Violence offered examples of promising violence prevention programs but prodded the staff of the funded programs to consider whether the requisite conditions were in place in their communities (The Colorado Trust, 2001).

5. Fairness might also require that the funder take into account the fact that different grantees come into an initiative with different levels of experience and organizational capacity.

6. The remaining two initiatives (CAHPI and VRSI) assumed that the applicant groups had carried out planning so as to prepare their applications.

7. In the Colorado Violence Prevention Initiative, The Colorado Trust contracted with two different consulting groups that provided grantees with two distinct forms of technical assistance: (a) content expertise on violence prevention and (b) coaching support on organizational development and group process issues (The Colorado Trust, 2001).

References

Arredondo, S., Aultman-Bettridge, T., Johnson, T. P., Williams, K. R., Ninneman, L., & Torp, K. (1999). *Preventing youth handgun violence: A national study with trends and patterns for the state of Colorado.* Boulder: University of Colorado, Center for the Study and Prevention of Violence.

Baker, Q., Davis, D. A., Gallerani, R., Sanchez, V., & Viadro, C. (2000). *An evaluation framework for community health programs.* Durham, NC: Center for the Advancement of Community-Based Public Health.

Benson, P. L. (1997). *All kids are our kids: What communities must do to raise caring and responsible children and adolescents.* San Francisco: Jossey-Bass.

Bracht, N. (Ed.) (1990). *Health promotion at the community level.* Newbury Park, CA: Sage.

Coleman, V., Holton, W. C., Olson, K., Robinson, S. C., & Morrison, T. (2001, January). Using knowledge and teamwork to reduce crime. *United States Attorneys' Bulletin,* pp. 11–19.

Connell, J. P., Kubisch, A. C., Schorr, L. B., & Weiss, C. H. (Eds.) (1995). *New approaches to evaluating community initiatives: Concepts, methods, and context.* Washington, DC: Aspen Institute.

Fawcett, S. B., Sterling, T. D., Paine-Andrews, A., Harris, K. J., Francisco, V. T., Richter, K. P., Lewis, R. K., & Schmid, T. L. (1995). *Evaluating community efforts to prevent cardiovascular diseases.* Atlanta, GA: Centers for Disease Control and Prevention, National Center for Chronic Disease Prevention and Health Promotion.

Fetterman, D., Kaftarian, S., & Wandersman, A. (Eds.) (1996). *Empowerment evaluation: Knowledge and tools for self-assessment and accountability.* Thousand Oaks, CA: Sage.

Fine, A. H., Thayer, C. E., & Coghlan, A. (1998). *Program evaluation practice in the nonprofit sector.* Washington, DC: Innovation Network.

Goodman, R. M., Speers, M. A., McLeroy, K. A., Fawcett, S., Kegler, M., Parker, E., Smith, S. R., Sterling, T. D., & Wallerstein, N. (1998). Identifying and defining the dimensions of community capacity to provide a basis for measurement. *Health Education and Behavior, 25,* 258–278.

Goodman, R., Wandersman, A., Chinman, M., Imm, P., & Morrissey, E. (1996). An ecological assessment of community-based interventions for prevention. *American Journal of Community Psychology, 24,* 33–61.

Gorin, S. S., & Arnold, J. (1998). *Health promotion handbook.* St. Louis, MO: C. V. Mosby.

Green, L. W., & Kreuter, M. W. (1990). *Health promotion planning: An educational and environmental approach* (2nd ed.). Palo Alto, CA: Mayfield.

Hawkins, J. D., & Catalano, R. F. (1992). *Communities that care.* San Francisco: Jossey-Bass.

Kennedy, D. M., Braga, A. A., & Piehl, A. M. (2001). *Developing and implementing Operation Ceasefire: Reducing gun violence.* Washington, DC: U.S. Department of Justice, National Institute of Justice.

Kreuter, M., & Lezin, N. (1998). *Are consortia/collaboratives effective in changing health status and health systems? A critical review of the literature.* Report prepared for the Office of Planning, Evaluation, and Legislation, Health Resources and Services Administration, Rockville, MD.

Kreuter, M. W., Lezin, N. A., Kreuter, M. W., & Green, L. W. (1998). *Community health promotion ideas that work: A field book for practitioners.* Sudbury, MA: Jones & Bartlett.

Linney, J. A., & Wandersman, A. (1991). *Prevention Plus III: Assessing alcohol and other drug prevention programs at the school and community level* (DHHS Publication No. (ADM)91–1817). Rockville, MD: U.S. Department of Health and Human Services, Office of Substance Abuse Prevention.

Milbank Memorial Fund. (1999). *New foundations in health: Six stories.* New York: Author.

Minkler, M. (Ed.). (1997). *Community organizing and community building for health.* New Brunswick, NJ: Rutgers University Press.

Morrissey, E., Wandersman, A., Seybolt, D., Nation, M., Crusto, C., & Davino, K. (1997). Toward a framework for bridging the gap between science and practice in prevention: A focus on evaluator and practitioner perspectives. *Evaluation and Program Planning, 20,* 367–377.

Oetting, E. R., & Beauvais, F. (1991). Critical incidents: Failure in prevention. *International Journal of the Addictions, 26,* 797–820.

Olds, D., Eckenrode, J., Henderson, C., Jr., Kitzman, H., Powers, J., Cole, R., Sidora, K., Morris, P., Pettitt, L.M., Luckey, D. (1997). Long term effects of home visitation on maternal life course and child abuse and neglect: Fifteen year follow-up of a randomized trial. *Journal of the American Medical Association, 278,* 637–643.

Patton, M. Q. (1997). *Utilization-focused evaluation: The new century text* (3rd ed.). Thousand Oaks, CA: Sage.

Posavac, E. J., & Carey, R. G. (1997). *Program evaluation: Methods and case studies* (5th ed.). Upper Saddle River, NJ: Prentice Hall.

Praeger, D. J. (1999). *Raising the value of philanthropy: A synthesis of informal interviews with foundation executives and observers of philanthropy.* Washington, DC: Grantmakers in Health.

Senge, P. (1990). *The fifth discipline: The art and practice of the learning organization.* New York: Doubleday.

Sievers, B., & Layton, T. (2000). Grantee/Grantor relations: Best of the worst practices. *Foundation News & Commentary, 41*(2), 30–37.

The Colorado Trust. (2001). *Building capacity for violence prevention: Executive summary of the final evaluation report on The Colorado Trust's Violence Prevention Initiative.* Denver, CO: Author.

W. K. Kellogg Foundation. (1998). *W. K. Kellogg Foundation evaluation handbook.* Battle Creek, MI: Author.

Wandersman, A., Morrissey, E., Davino, K., Seybolt, D., Crusto, C., Nation, M., Goodman, R., & Imm, P. (1998). Comprehensive quality programming and accountability: Eight essential strategies for implementing successful prevention programs. *Journal of Primary Prevention, 19*(1), 3–30.

Weiss, C. H. (1995). Nothing as practical as good theory: Exploring theory-based evaluation for comprehensive community initiatives for children and families. In J. P. Connell, A. C. Kubisch, L. B. Schorr, & C. H. Weiss (Eds.), *New approaches to evaluating community initiatives: Concepts, methods, and context* (pp. 65–92). Washington, DC: Aspen Institute.

Wholey, J. S. (1994). Assessing the feasibility and likely usefulness of evaluation. In J. S. Wholey, H. P. Hatry, & K. E. Newcomer (Eds.), *Handbook of practical program evaluation* (pp. 15–19). San Francisco: Jossey-Bass.

Index

About the Editors

Douglas V. Easterling, Ph.D., is Director of the Division for Community-Based Evaluation within the Center for the Study of Social Issues at the University of North Carolina at Greensboro. Through the division, he has served as the principal investigator on evaluations of the Winston-Salem Foundation's initiative to build social capital and the Z. Smith Reynolds Foundation's initiative to improve race relations. He has also assisted the Community Foundation of Greater Greensboro, the Warner Foundation, the Mary Reynolds Babcock Foundation, and The Conservation Fund in designing evaluation systems and clarifying program intent. From 1992 to 1999, he served as the director of research and evaluation at The Colorado Trust. In that capacity, he commissioned evaluations of the foundation's initiatives (including the seven initiatives described in this book) and facilitated the foundation's process of learning from the results. He has published articles and books on the topics of program evaluation, community-based health promotion, and nuclear waste policy. He also teaches the evaluation module for the Health Forum's fellowship programs, and he served on the CENTERED Blue Ribbon Panel that was convened by the Centers for Disease Control and Prevention to improve the evaluation of projects that aim to reduce racial/ethnic disparities in health. In February 2002, he delivered the Fischer Francis Trees & Watts Keynote Address at the Community Trust Conference in New Zealand. He holds a Ph.D. in public policy and management from the University of Pennsylvania, an M.A. in quantitative psychology from the University of North Carolina at Chapel Hill, and a B.A. from Carleton College.

Kaia M. Gallagher, Ph.D., is Director of Evaluation and Manager for the Center for Research Strategies, a research and evaluation consulting firm in Denver, Colorado. With more than 25 years of experience, she currently serves as the evaluator for a number of federal, state, and local programs, focusing in particular on the effectiveness of prevention programs designed to change the risk behaviors of youth. Her career focus has been on promoting the use of strategically collected information to enhance the development and performance of programs in the health, education, and social service sectors. In this capacity, she provides consulting services in the areas of strategic planning, needs assessment, outcome evaluations, and development of outcome assessment tools. She also develops business plans that disseminate research models into marketable products and services. Previously, she worked in a number of evaluation offices within the U.S. Department of Health and Human Services (DHHS), including the Office of the Assistant Secretary for Planning and Evaluation. She currently provides evaluation services to DHHS programs funded by the Centers for Disease Control and Prevention, the Office of Adolescent Pregnancy and Parenting, the Family Youth and Services Bureau, and the Health Resources and Services Administration. She is Assistant Clinical Professor in the Department of Preventive Medicine and Biometrics within the University of Colorado Health Sciences Center. She is a member of the board of directors for the National Organization of Adolescent Pregnancy, Parenting, and Prevention. She earned her Ph.D. in sociology from Brown University.

Dora G. Lodwick, Ph.D., founded the REFT Institute, which focuses on research, evaluation, facilitation, and training, in Centennial, Colorado. She has evaluated programs and other initiatives in the areas of participatory community-based development, leadership development, health, immigrants and refugees, aging, and environmental impacts. She has published in several of those areas for more than 20 years. She has worked extensively in Latin America, and she speaks Portuguese and Spanish. She has been a university professor for 15 years at Miami University of Ohio, Oregon State University, and the University of Denver, where she established the master's degree program in applied social research and evaluation. She has served the Society for Applied Sociology (SAS) as president, as a board member, and in other capacities and has represented SAS on the Commission on Applied and Clinical Sociology. She has also held leadership positions in the American Sociological Association.

About the Contributors

James V. Adams-Berger, M.A., is President of OMNI Research and Training and OMNI Institute and has worked for these companies since 1992. His primary technical areas of expertise include survey development, program evaluation, and both qualitative and quantitative data analysis. He has served as the principal investigator for a number of research and evaluation projects with a wide range of focus areas, including suicide prevention, childhood immunization, community development, school dropout prevention, and substance abuse.

Ross F. Conner, Ph.D., is Director of the Center for Community Health Research at the University of California, Irvine. He received his Ph.D. and M.A. from Northwestern University (social psychology/evaluation) and his B.A. from Johns Hopkins University. His research focuses on community health promotion/disease prevention programs. Currently, he is the principal investigator for the ACCT Project: Achieving Cancer Control Together With Koreans and Chinese in Orange County (California), a multiyear collaborative effort involving the university and three community-based groups. He is also collaborating with other community colleagues on an HIV prevention program for Spanish-speaking Latino men. His recent work on the Colorado Healthy Communities Initiative (described in this book) received the American Evaluation Association's 2002 Outstanding Evaluation Award. He is the author or coauthor of nine books and numerous articles. He is the past president of the American Evaluation Association. He also works with various foundations, government agencies, and organizations on evaluation and community health issues.

Marc B. Davidson completed his undergraduate work at the University of California, San Diego, and the University of California, Berkeley, in the areas of anthropology and psychology. His graduate work in health psychology and community health at the School of Social Ecology at the University of California, Irvine, involved research in the areas of program evaluation and health promotion. He also has been extensively involved in community health initiatives outside of the university environment. Combining a formal education in health psychology with patient care experience as an emergency medic, he has presented chronic illness management talks to counseling psychologists, nurses, and patients, with an emphasis on effective day-to-day coping skills. In addition, he has planned and promoted events for the American Diabetes Association and has conducted publicity campaigns for medical symposia.

Catherine L. Dempsey, Ph.D., is Senior Instructor in the Division of Substance Abuse within the Department of Psychiatry at the University of Colorado School of Medicine. She received her B.S. in psychology and M.P.H. in health administration from Emory University and recently received her Ph.D. in health and behavioral sciences from the University of Colorado. Currently, she is a co-investigator and node coordinator for the National Institute on Drug Abuse Clinical Trials Network, Rocky Mountain Node, a research grant investigating the differential efficacy of various treatments for substance abuse in diverse populations. She has several years of experience in implementing community-based research in diverse populations. Her areas of expertise include psychiatric epidemiology, psychiatric assessments, cross-cultural community-based research, posttraumatic stress disorder, and substance abuse in diverse populations.

Jodi G. Drisko is Director of Survey Research and Evaluation in Health Statistics for the Colorado Department of Public Health and Environment. She received her M.S.P.H. in 1994 from the University of Colorado Health Sciences Center. She worked from 1993 to 1999 evaluating The Colorado Trust's Teen Pregnancy Prevention 2000 Initiative, conducting needs assessments for the Ryan White Title I and II programs, and researching barriers to prenatal care for teens. From 1999 to June 2002, she managed the quality improvement and program evaluation department for Denver Health's Community Health Services. She has years of experience in data analysis, assessment, performance improvement, and program evaluation.

Donna K. Duffy, M.A., was project director of the Colorado School Health Education Initiative (described in this book) for 6 years and has worked extensively with school districts throughout the United States in the area of health education. She provides technical assistance and professional staff development to school personnel in the areas of school/community partnerships, health education curriculum selection and implementation, and health education staff/committee development. She also works with school boards to support health education.

Jill A. Elnicki, M.P.H., is Evaluation Consultant with the Rocky Mountain Center for Health Promotion and Education (RMC), a national training and technical assistance center focused on school health programming. She joined the RMC team in 1995, serving as an evaluation liaison to the Colorado School

Health Education Initiative (described in this book). Currently, she oversees evaluation of RMC projects and provides technical assistance to school districts and other youth-serving agencies in the areas of program evaluation, tobacco use prevention and reduction, and standards-based health education. Prior to her years at RMC, she worked at the Colorado Department of Public Health and Environment in community health education and in the Division of Epidemiology at the University of Minnesota.

Douglas H. Fernald, M.A., is Professional Research Assistant in the Department of Family Medicine at the University of Colorado Health Sciences Center. He received an M.A. in medical anthropology from the University of Colorado, Denver, and a B.A. in history and political science from Colorado College. He has expertise in research and evaluation using qualitative research methods, including research design, instrument design, interviewing, data analysis, and qualitative data analysis software. His research interests include improving care for medically underserved populations, improving patient safety, examining the role of the family in medical decision making, and using innovative qualitative research and evaluation methods.

Peggy L. Hill, M.S., works for Rocky Mountain Institute, an entrepreneurial nonprofit creating a more secure, prosperous, and life-sustaining planet. She is a curious observer of living systems and the ways in which individuals learn and behave. She sees humans as semiconscious but powerful actors within those systems, and she believes that nature will become an increasingly severe teacher on many levels unless we soon learn a bit of humility. She earned graduate degrees in agronomy and education from Purdue University, where she studied the ecology of agriculture, human development, and community organization. Over the past 20 years, she has developed and managed a variety of programs in vulnerable and marginalized populations. While at the University of Colorado Health Sciences Center, and with the support of The Colorado Trust, she applied the concept of a learning group to assist family service workers and their supervisors to engage in reflective practice and program improvement.

Michelle Miller Kobayashi, M.S.P.H., is Vice President of National Research Center. She has a master's degree in public health with an emphasis on epidemiology and biostatistics. She has designed and overseen a wide variety of research and evaluation projects on topics such as after-school programming and positive youth development, palliative care, obesity prevention, domestic violence, rural mental health service provision, health care access, and community performance measurement. She has worked extensively on outcome assesssment in cancer, speech and audiology, biofeedback, and asthma. She coauthored (with Thomas I. Miller) *Citizen Surveys: How to Do Them, How to Use Them, What They Mean.*

Deborah S. Main, Ph.D., a social psychologist, is Director of the Behavioral Sciences Core in the Colorado Health Outcomes Program and Associate Professor in the Department of Family Medicine at the University of Colorado Health Sciences Center. She has more than 15 years of experience in behavioral and practice-based research with a particular interest in understanding the individual and organizational features that affect the uptake and outcomes of health and health care interventions. She is also the research director of the Agency for Healthcare Research and Quality-funded Colorado Research Network (CaReNet), a practice-based research organization consisting of 18 primary care practices and more than 250 clinicians dedicated to understanding the health and health care issues of disadvantaged populations. She has considerable experience in both qualitative and quantitative methods of data collection and analysis. She has been the principal investigator on two large funded studies that used mixed methods of data collection to understand the adoption, implementation, and realistic impact of health education interventions in school and community settings.

Thomas I. Miller has worked in state and local government since 1977, founding National Research Center in 1994. He received a Ph.D. in research and evaluation methods from the University of Colorado. He has designed, overseen, and written results of hundreds of research projects and has presented his findings to a wide variety of audiences (both academic and lay). He has written about survey research in journals devoted to public management, including *Public Administration Review, Journal of the American Planning Association, Journal of Policy Analysis and Management, Management Science,* and *Policy Analysis and Governing.* He also was cofounder of Evaluation Systems International, a health care outcome research and software company. He also has published in a variety of health care journals and is coauthor of *Benefits of Psychotherapy,* a book reporting the results of the first meta-analysis.

John R. Moran, Jr. serves as president and chief executive officer of The Colorado Trust, a grantmaking foundation dedicated to advancing the health and well-being of the people of Colorado. In this capacity, Moran represents the interests of The Trust in the community as well as regionally and nationally, leads (in his words) "a most competent staff" of program officers, evaluators and financial administrators, and serves as an *ex-officio* member of the Board of Trustees. Before being named president of The Colorado Trust in 1991, Moran served as legal counsel to The Trust from the time of its founding in 1985. From 1958 to 1991, he was a practicing attorney in Denver representing, among others, health-care-related clients and foundations. Moran also served as a member of the Colorado House of Representatives, and as a commissioned officer on active duty with the U.S. Navy. He received a bachelor of laws degree in 1955 and a doctor of laws degree in 1970, both from the

University of Denver. In 1952, he earned his undergraduate degree from the University of Notre Dame. Moran is an active member of many civic and professional organizations, and a frequent speaker on issues affecting foundations.

Kathryn A. Judge Nearing, M.A., is Senior Research Associate at OMNI Research and Training and OMNI Institute. Her responsibilities include instrument development, qualitative consultation, project management, and grant writing. Her projects include the evaluation of the Assets for Colorado Youth Initiative (she leads project components exploring integration of the Asset framework/philosophy at the organizational and personal levels, the spread and reach of the Asset movement in Colorado, and Asset Champions), the evaluation of a Colorado Trust-funded initiative to prevent suicide through school-based intervention, the evaluation of the Daniels Fund's first year of grant making, and a needs assessment for Jewish Family Service of Colorado focused on assessing the needs of individuals living with disabilities and their family members in the Jewish community. She also serves as a qualitative consultant for Prevention Evaluation Partners, an evaluation system supporting substance abuse prevention block grant providers funded by Colorado's Alcohol and Drug Abuse Division.

Gabriela Robles, M.A., has more than 10 years of experience working on community health efforts in different capacities. Most recently, for the past 3 years, she was the program officer at the St. Joseph Health System Foundation in Orange, California. In this capacity, she led health system efforts to benefit the economically poor and to promote healthy community efforts. In addition, she has worked for several health-related nonprofit organizations in Southern California. She has worked directly with monolingual immigrant communities and has conducted numerous community trainings on health promotion and advocacy. She has a master's degree in urban and regional planning, with an emphasis on community-based planning for health, from the University of California, Irvine.

Sora Park Tanjasiri, Dr.P.H., M.P.H., is Researcher in the School of Social Ecology at the University of California, Irvine. Her work focuses on the community health needs of diverse populations, including both physical health and community capacity building. For 3 years, she has participated in the evaluation of the Colorado Healthy Communities Initiative (described in this book) and examined the ways in which community coalitions have improved the individual capacities, community collaborations, and health outcomes of their citizens. She is especially interested in the concerns of Asian Americans and Pacific Islanders, and her current projects include the evaluation of cancer prevention and early detection efforts among Cambodians, Chamorros, Chinese, Hmong, Koreans, Laotians, Samoans, Thais, Tongans, and Vietnamese throughout California. In addition to her professional work, she serves as an adviser to numerous nonprofit community organizations and coalitions. She received her degrees in community health sciences from the School of Public Health at the University of California, Los Angeles.

Carolyn J. Tressler, M.S.P.H., has worked in the area of research and program evaluation for 15 years, including several community-based health promotion initiatives. She received an M.S. in public health in 1988 from the University of Colorado Health Sciences Center. Her areas of interest and expertise include instrument development, interview survey design, focus group development, and qualitative analysis. Populations of particular interest to her include the medically underserved, refugee families, and adolescents.

Allan Wallis, Ph.D., is Associate Professor of Public Policy in the Graduate School of Public Affairs at the University of Colorado at Denver, where he directs the Ph.D. program in public affairs. His principal areas of research are regional governance and growth management. His current work on regionalism is being funded by the MacArthur Foundation. He is the author of *Wheel Estate: The Rise and Decline of Mobile Homes.* He holds a Ph.D. in environmental psychology from the City University of New York, a master's in public administration from Harvard University, and a bachelor's of architecture from the Cooper Union. He has taught architecture at the University of Colorado and at Ball State University. He has also taught urban design and town planning at the Pratt Institute and the Cooper Union.